REHABILITATION OF THE SEVERELY BRAIN-INJURED ADULT

A Practical Approach

THERAPY IN PRACTICE

Series Editor: Jo Campling

This series of books is aimed at 'therapists' concerned with rehabilitation in a very broad sense. The intended audience particularly includes occupational therapists, physiotherapists and speech therapists, but many titles will also be of interest to nurses, psychologists, medical staff, social workers, teachers or volunteer workers. Some volumes will be interdisciplinary, others aimed at one particular profession. All titles will be comprehensive but concise, and practical but with due reference to relevant theory and evidence. They are not research monographs but focus on professional practice, and will be of value to both students and qualified personnel.

Titles Available

'Communication Problems in Elderly People' *Rosemary Gravell*
'Occupational Therapy for Children with Disabilities' *Dorothy E. Penso*
'Living Skills for Mentally Handicapped People' *Christine Peck and Chia Swee Hong*
'Physiotherapy and the Elderly Patient' *Paul Wagstaff and Davis Coakley*

Titles in Preparation

'Modern Electrotherapy' *Christopher Hayne*
'Assessment of Physically Disabled People at Home' *Kathleen Maczka*
'Occupational Therapy Practice in Psychiatry' *Linda Finlay*
'Movement Exercises for Language Difficulties' *M. Nash-Wortham*
'Management in Occupational Therapy' *Zielfa B. Maslin*
'Community Occupational Therapy with Mentally Handicapped People' *Debbie Isaac*
'Understanding Dysphasia' *Lesley Jordan and Rita Twiston Davies*
'Psychology in Physiotherapy' *Cynthia Fox*
'Working with Bilingual Language Disability' *Edited by Deirdre M. Duncan*
'Rehabilitation of the Older Patient' *Edited by Amanda J. Squires*

REHABILITATION OF THE SEVERELY BRAIN-INJURED ADULT

A Practical Approach

Edited by Ian Fussey and Gordon Muir Giles

WITHDRAWN

London   Sydney
CROOM HELM

First published in 1988 by
Croom Helm Ltd
11 New Fetter Lane, London EC4P 4EE

Croom Helm Australia
44–50 Waterloo Road, North Ryde
2113, New South Wales

Distributed exclusively in the USA and non-exclusively in Canada by
Paul H. Brookes Publishing Co., Post Office Box 10624, Baltimore,
Maryland 21285

Printed in Great Britain by
St. Edmundsbury Press Ltd
Bury St. Edmunds, Suffolk

ISBN 0 7099 4904 9

British Library Cataloguing in Publication Data

Rehabilitation of the severely brain-injured
    adult : a practical approach. — (Therapy
    in practice).
    1. Brain damage — Patients —
    Rehabilitation
    I. Fussey, Ian II. Giles, Gordon Muir
    III. Series
    362.1′968   RC386.2

    ISBN 0–7099–4904–9

Contents

Contributors

Paul Burgess, BA
Research Officer, Medical Research Council, Applied Psychology Unit, Cambridge, UK

Jo Clark-Wilson, BA, DipCOT
Senior Occupational Therapist, The Kemsley Unit, St. Andrew's Hospital, Northampton, UK

John Cumberpatch, RMN
Charge Nurse, The Kemsley Unit, St. Andrew's Hospital, Northampton, UK

Jill Edney, CertEd
Teacher, The Kemsley Unit, St. Andrew's Hospital, Northampton, UK

Ann Gent, MCSP
Superintendent Physiotherapist, The Kemsley Unit, St. Andrew's Hospital, Northampton, UK

Claire Grant, RMN
Sister, The Kemsley Unit, St. Andrew's Hospital, Northampton, UK

Jennifer Hooper-Roe, MCSP
Formerly: Senior Physiotherapist, The Kemsley Unit, St. Andrew's Hospital, Northampton, UK

Mary Lees, AIMSW
Principal Social Worker, The Kemsley Unit, St. Andrew's Hospital, Northampton, UK

Carmella Mazzella-Gordon, MS, CCC
Formerly: Speech and Language Pathologist, in private practice, Danville, California, USA

Martyn Rose, FRCS
Consultant, The Kemsley Unit, St. Andrew's Hospital, Northampton, UK

Kelley L. Wicks, MS
Speech Pathologist, Berkeley, California, USA

Rodger Ll. Wood, PhD, ABPsS
Director of Brain Injury Rehabilitation Services, Casa Colina Hospital for Rehabilitation Medicine, Pomona, California, USA, and Honorary Research Fellow, Institute of Health Care Studies, University College, Swansea, UK

THE EDITORS

Ian Fussey, MSc, ABPsS
Consultant Psychologist, The Leicester Clinic, Leicester, UK. *Formerly*: Principal Clinical Psychologist, The Kemsley Unit, St. Andrew's Hospital, Northampton, UK

Gordon Muir Giles, BA, DipCOT, OTR
Clinical Director, Transitions: Bay Area Head Injury Recovery Center, Berkeley, California 94705, USA

Introduction

This book centres around the work of a group of individuals who have, at one time or another, been therapists at the Kemsley Unit, St. Andrew's Hospital, Northampton, England. Although a content analysis of the following pages would no doubt reveal that 'behaviour' is one of the most frequently used words, behaviourism is only part of the philosophy of these workers. It is a sad fact that post-acute brain injury rehabilitation falls beyond the margins of mainstream clinical practice. Most research in the area of brain injury is either directed at the acute patient or is descriptive in nature. The negative attitude widely held about post-acute treatment is matched by the scarcity of resources with which to pursue it, so that to many it remains a non-issue, never entering the realm of serious discussion. A report of the Royal College of Physicians, entitled *Physical Disability in 1986 and Beyond*, describes the present crisis in the provision of care, treatment and rehabilitation for the head-injured. It is estimated that approximately 7500 major head injuries occur annually in England and Wales, and that the prevalence of serious head injury disability is probably about 150 per 100,000 population. In the United States the scope of the problem is immense. In 1974 some 422,000 new cases occurred, a rate of 200 new head injuries per 100,000 population per year (Anderson and McLaurin, 1980). There are a number of reasons for examining the question of efficacy of post-acute treatment more energetically.

Firstly, the problems of the severely impaired brain-injured do not go away, and in some cases become worse through time, possibly due to inappropriate new learning. This constitutes an immense human cost for the patients and their carers — often the patient's family.

Secondly, although there is considerable evidence relating to improvement in outcome associated with better surgical management in the hours and days after injury, the effectiveness of early intensive rehabilitation is unclear. All those who do not die or enter a persistent vegetative state get better to some degree. This spontaneous recovery so complicates research that any benefits of early intervention over more conservative management have not been demonstrated. This is at least partly due to the fact that available means of measuring outcome are so gross that the effects of therapy would have to be very dramatic before they would be evident.

The position with the post-acute patient is more clear-cut. Improvement as a result of treatment is far easier to demonstrate due to the absence of spontaneous recovery. This opens the possibility of taking information gained from post-acute treatment and applying this knowledge to the acute stage. Also, with increasing evidence of the effectiveness of post-acute interventions it should lead us to examine carefully how to allocate resources to the best advantage. Whatever the most appropriate mix of resources for acute and post-acute care, the current situation, in which the patient is often abandoned after 'failing to respond to therapy', is surely inappropriate. A more holistic approach providing care, support and therapy, depending on the needs of the patient, is overdue.

A NOTE ON TERMINOLOGY

Although a distinction between closed and penetrating brain injury may be useful for research it does not coincide with the distribution of patients in a busy rehabilitation unit. In these pages, since we are more interested in the effects of brain injury and its treatment than in its cause, the definition used is wider than those more frequently adopted. This has the disadvantage of imprecision, but the advantage of being more like the real world as experienced by most therapists and at least touching on the treatment of patients whose conditions would otherwise be rarely mentioned. Here brain injury is defined as the result of an insult to the brain causing permanent damage which is usually confirmable on nuclear magnetic resonance imaging. Brain injury may be due to:

(1) Trauma — closed or open. Closed-head injury is the result of a brain being subjected to forces of acceleration and deceleration within a rigid skull, leading to diffuse and widespread axonal shearing, the location of which depends on the anatomical structure of brain tissue. Open (or penetrating) brain injury involves penetration of the skull and the membranes surrounding the brain by a foreign object such as a projectile, as in a gunshot

wound. Only in rare cases (such as when the skull is completely immobilised) is a penetrating injury not associated with some diffuse axonal shearing.

(2) Infections such as herpes simplex encephalitis.

(3) Metabolic disturbances such as anoxia, ischaemia or hypoglycaemia.

(4) Vascular damage such as aneurysms.

Various symptom complexes are associated with different pathologies. The central focus of this book is traumatic brain injury. Patients with other diagnoses are discussed where their treatment is of particular interest. Discussion is limited to adults, due to the complexity of the issues involved in the interaction of development and damage. Work conducted with an already mature nervous system is simpler to evaluate. Authors were asked to limit case discussion to a small number of patients, and where possible the same patients are described from a variety of therapist perspectives. The reader should note that this is not designed as a textbook and the authors could not hope to cover the full range of approaches available to the therapist working with brain injury. The approaches detailed here may be idiosyncratic, but it is hoped that this may serve to stimulate thought.

From this book the reader should gain the understanding that:

(1) rehabilitation techniques can be applied with success even in the most severe cases of brain injury;

(2) a behavioural approach can help patients maximise their functional ability despite relatively fixed cognitive deficits;

(3) behaviour disorders need not be a barrier to effective rehabilitation;

(4) a behaviour therapy approach can provide a model for interdisciplinary practice.

Acknowledgements

We wish to thank all those who have guided our thinking and helped us in the preparation of this book. Special acknowledgement must go to Peter Eames, who masterminded the Kemsley Unit for six years and who is now at Burden Neurological Institute, Bristol. His influence is present throughout the book. As editors we of course wish to thank our contributors, some of whom commented on chapters not their own. Special thanks are due to Paul Burgess BA. Thanks are also due to Liz Allen MS, Paul Bach-y-Rita MD, Richard Balliet PhD, Christine Cordle MSc, Carmella Gordon MA, Harry Hatzichristidis BA, Randy Larquin BA, Michael Shore PhD and Rodger Wood PhD, all of whom read and commented on earlier versions of parts of this manuscript. However, any errors of interpretation remain the responsibility of the authors.

IAN FUSSEY
Northampton, UK

GORDON MUIR GILES
Berkeley, California, USA

1

Models of Brain Injury Rehabilitation: From Theory to Practice

Gordon Muir Giles and Ian Fussey

Patients requiring rehabilitation after severe brain injury can display a wide range of deficits. Marked cognitive, physical, behavioural, medical and psychiatric sequelae are common and may result in severe functional disabilities. Unfortunately the services available to this group of patients are frequently inadequate in both Great Britain and the USA (Gloag, 1985a). The more severely handicapped the patients, the harder they are to place. Such patients often live for long periods in grossly inadequate settings such as psychiatric or mental handicap hospitals or in acute surgical wards, and are impossible to discharge long after the need for acute care ends (Evans *et al.*, 1981; Acton, 1982; Eames and Wood, 1985a).

Central to the problem is not only lack of resources but also the absence of any shared philosophy or common orientation towards rehabilitation of the severely brain-injured adult. Therapists must choose between a number of competing models, all with differing implications for therapy. Controversy continues as to what constitutes adequate and appropriate treatment: Should treatment be applied early or late? Can prognosis be determined and how? Is therapy effective and how long should it be continued?

As a result of this fundamental lack of agreement patients undergo fragmented approaches to rehabilitation. The model presented in this book is that of behaviour therapy, which has a number of advantages. It is a well-established and widely used methodology fostering research and a problem-solving approach to maladaptive behaviours. Case methodologies in behaviour therapy offer paradigms for evaluation and treatment, as well as providing a model for rehabilitation of the brain-injured and a uniform approach between staff.

SEVERITY OF BRAIN INJURY

Severity of brain injury refers to the amount of damage the brain has incurred through trauma. Since the brain cannot be examined directly, severity is usually inferred from the extent and duration of alterations in responsiveness. It should be recognised, however, that this type of assessment does not take into account focal damage where a small area of damage can have significant effects on function. The fact that diffuse and focal damage frequently occur together may obscure the importance of the focal damage. It is important to distinguish severity of injury from severity of outcome (Rose, 1980). A number of scales have been developed to assess the status of the acutely brain-injured patient (Teasdale and Jennett, 1974; Brinkmann et al., 1976) which can be useful in charting progress and in the early detection of complications. Other scales look at outcome (Smith et al., 1979) and there have been frequent attempts made to relate the two (Jennett et al., 1981; Rappaport et al., 1982; Hall et al., 1985).

Methods used to assess the severity of brain injury in the acute stages have developed rapidly over the past 20 years. A number of scales have been developed; the best-known of which is the Glasgow Coma Scale. In the very acute stages where the issues involved are essentially binary — on one hand death or a persisting vegetative state, and on the other hand, survival — there are some fairly robust indicators such as impaired pupillary reaction, impaired eye movements (oculocephalic reflex), abnormal motor responses, increased intracranial pressure, and paradoxical arousal (Becker et al., 1977). The type of intracranial lesion also has implications for outcome (Gennarelli et al., 1982; Seelig et al., 1981).

Even here, however, where predictive power is strongest there are individual exceptions. Persistent vegetative state (PVS) may in some cases resolve into some higher level of cognitive function (Berrol, 1986; Jennett and Teasdale, 1981; Arts et al., 1985). There remains no absolute measure of severity of brain injury, and views vary as to how it should be defined (Jennett and Teasdale, 1981). Duration of coma and length of post-traumatic amnesia (PTA) are the most accepted criteria. Severe brain injury has been defined as leading to coma in excess of 6 hours or to PTA in excess of 24 hours (Jennett and Teasdale, 1981; Russell and Smith, 1961). Mild and moderate head injury are variously defined, but below this level. Duration of coma and length of PTA are correlated, and are both good indicators of severity of brain trauma. Age is an important factor predictive of good outcome: children and adolescents show better outcomes than adults with similar injuries (Berger et al., 1985; Jennett et al., 1977).

Jennett and Teasdale (1981) have related PTA to outcome at six months using the Glasgow Outcome Scale (GOS) (Jennett and Bond, 1975). Although there is a clear trend in the group data, indicating that the longer the PTA the worse the likely outcome, the trend is far too weak to make firm predictions in any *individual* case. Only by using few (and therefore gross) outcome categories can a reasonable level of predictive power be maintained. Although one of the aims of producing this type of predictive tool has been to assess comparative effectiveness of treatment methods (Evans et al., 1981; Hall et al., 1985), it is difficult to accept that a measure as imprecise as GOS could be used for such a purpose. Recognition of the limitations of the GOS have led to the attempt to produce more sensitive measures (Hall et al., 1985). Assessment schedules for the brain-injured have a number of purposes unrelated to prediction. The Glasgow Assessment Schedule (GAS) presents a comprehensive rating which includes the assessment of physical, psychological, social, personality and activities of daily living (ADL) deficits (Livingston and Livingston, 1985) and could be used to note trends in recovery and responses to interventions.

A related issue is the length of the recovery processes. Until recently it was widely believed that significant recovery of function occurs exclusively in the first six months to a year following injury. This view has been supported by a series of studies by Jennett's group in Glasgow (Jennett and Teasdale, 1981) but can now be contrasted with a number of studies demonstrating continued improvement beyond this period. This has been shown to be irrespective of treatment methods (Levin et al., 1979; Hall et al., 1985) and a handful of studies have demonstrated treatment effect well beyond a period of spontaneous recovery (Prigatano et al., 1984; Eames and Wood, 1985a). To some extent these differences in findings may reflect the inadequate sensitivity of the assessment instruments producing research artefacts (Hall et al., 1985) and discounted non-significant findings (Levin et al., 1979). Much of the disagreement may also be due to choice of assessment domain.

3

Results of neuropsychological testing may stabilise well before findings on measures of community living skills. When the period of rapid spontaneous improvement is complete, energetic therapeutic intervention can play a vital role in helping patients achieve better social adjustment and in developing appropriate adaptation to disability despite relatively fixed neuropsychological deficits.

While someone with a severe brain injury may achieve an apparently full recovery, an individual with a 'mild' brain injury may show continuing problems (Colohan et al., 1986). Mild brain injuries are usually defined as injuries with loss of consciousness for less than 20 minutes or a Glasgow coma score of 13–15 (Rimel et al., 1981; Colohan et al., 1986). Controversy remains as to whether the long-term problems found in patients who have sustained apparently minor injury are organic in nature, and a link has often been made between the so-called 'post-concussion syndrome' (PCS) and claims for financial compensation (Miller, 1961, 1966; Merskey and Woodforde, 1972; Cartlidge, 1978). The symptoms most frequently associated with PCS are problems with memory, increased fatigue, irritability, anxiety, dizziness and headaches. Rimel et al. (1981) examined 424 patients three months after they had incurred a minor brain injury defined as unconsciousness of 20 minutes or less. Of these 424 patients 79 per cent complained of persistent headaches, and 59 per cent described problems with their memory. Of those patients who had been employed before the accident, 34 per cent were unemployed three months later. Most patients were found to be normal on neurological examination but showed persisting deficits in attention, concentration and memory. Litigation and compensation were described as having a minimal role in determining outcome, and the stress caused by persisting symptoms was highlighted as a significant factor in the long-term disability of these patients. In a more recent and better-controlled study Dikman et al. (1986) compared 20 subjects with mild head injuries with an uninjured control group at one month and one year after injury on a battery of neuropsychological and psychosocial measures. In contrast to the Rimel et al. study, results indicated that a single mild head injury in an individual with no prior compromising condition is associated with only mild difficulties one month post-injury. Continuing problems are associated with orthopaedic and soft tissue injuries. This study would have benefited from an orthopaedic control group, and the actual number of patients followed is small.

When the Rimel and Dikman studies are considered together they may indicate that minor injuries are likely to be more significant when they are repeated (accumulative effect) and when they occur in an individual who is already neurologically compromised. In Rimel's study 31 per cent of patients in their large series had a prior brain injury. Van Zomeren and co-workers (1984) have suggested that the mildly brain-injured may feel under considerable stress in having to cope with reduced memory, attention and information-processing capacities; stresses which do not apply to the more severely brain-injured (Fordyce et al., 1985). A number of workers have used radiological techniques such as CT scans to look for evidence of brain damage after mild brain injury. Findings indicate that even where patients remain asymptomatic, brain damage may have occurred (see Binder, 1986, for a review). The existence of post-concussional symptoms in the severely brain-injured suggests an organic aetiology (McKinlay et al., 1983). Although the issue of financial compensation should not be discounted, the organic consequences of mild brain trauma may well have been underestimated in the past (Jennett and Teasdale, 1981).

This is shown by the cumulative effect of mild brain trauma. Gronwall and Wrightson (1975) found that patients with a history of previous head trauma recovered more slowly than patients without such a history. Similarly the severity of cerebral atrophy found in professional boxers increased in relation to their number of fights (Casson et al., 1982). Patients over 40 are more likely to have persisting symptoms than patients under 30 (Denker, 1944) and there is recent evidence linking mild brain injury to Alzheimer's disease. Mild injuries may also have significant effects when they coexist with other types of trauma such as spinal cord injuries (Davidoff et al., 1985a,b).

Drawing attention to the limitations and complications of attempting to predict outcome should not be taken to suggest that such attempts will ultimately prove to be of doubtful value. It should serve to underline the limitations of prognostication, and should emphasise the fact that assessment of outcome must depend on measures which clearly relate to the disabilities of the individual patient (Brooks et al., 1986).

5

FAMILY AND SOCIAL CONSEQUENCES OF BRAIN INJURY

A significant proportion of the severely brain-injured retain physical, cognitive and behavioural impairments serious enough to prevent them from living fully independent lives. Some remain almost totally dependent. Other forms of severe physical trauma leave the individual cognitively intact and more able to adjust to reduced ability. In the brain-injured, however, the ability to compensate is limited as a result of the damage itself. This is particularly tragic as brain injury is most frequent among adolescents and young adults who had hopes and expectations which are now unlikely to be fulfilled. The fact that the individual may have no memory for the injury, and for a considerable amount of the recovery process, complicates accommodation to the new handicapped state. Unlike stroke patients, who are frequently older and already possess established social networks providing care and support, the young brain-injured patient is often socially isolated. Studies which have examined the effect of a brain injury on the patient's family have been consistent in their findings that cognitive impairments and personality changes are more difficult for families to cope with than physical impairments (Bond, 1975; Thomsen, 1974; Weddell et al., 1980). Parents may be better able than spouses to tolerate change in the patient (Thomsen, 1974) but none the less may go through a considerable period of grieving for the greatly changed family member. It may be considerably easier for parents to adjust to the increased level of dependence of the severely brain-injured because a high level of dependency was experienced with the individual in childhood. Weddell et al. (1980) demonstrated that only a small proportion of severely brain-injured adults were able to return to their former employment. Nearly 50 per cent were unable to work at all, and in half of these cases care was provided by parents. One or both of the parents may have given up work to look after patients who were heavily dependent.

Oddy and co-workers (1978) examined stress in relatives of brain-injured patients. Expressed stress level was influenced by the relative's perception of personality changes and subjective deficits. It was not affected by the severity of brain injury, nor by whether patients had resumed work. Relatives' complaints highlighted what they saw as poor communication from professionals. Relatives often felt that they were not given sufficient information about the extent and nature of injury, a finding which is consistent with the results of a number of earlier studies (Thomsen, 1974; Panting and Merry, 1972). Personality change in the brain-injured has been found to be far more significant than other factors in causing families stress (Lezak, 1978; Brooks and McKinlay, 1983). Problems may relate to the patient's reduced capacity for social perceptiveness which can result in self-centred behaviour and lack of insight. Lack of self-control and impulsivity, as well as memory problems, can lead to a greatly reduced ability to plan and carry out actions. The patient may be disinhibited, leading to behaviour which the family find both disgusting and embarrassing. Sexual behaviours may be either greatly increased or absent (Miller *et al.*, 1986). Altered emotional responsiveness is frequently a problem, with apathy, silliness and increased touching being reported as common problems.

Families may also feel trapped and isolated, and may be in physical danger from the brain-injured person. Young children find the presence of a 'changed' father or mother particularly difficult. Spouses may have particular problems because of ambivalent feelings towards a markedly changed individual. Spouses often feel guilty about resenting the demands placed upon them by patient care, further isolating them from family and friends. Unfortunately it is often automatically assumed that the patient will go home after the patient has 'ceased to make progress' at the rehabilitation setting. Family members may need to be more involved in decisions concerning discharge and placement. While it is reasonable to encourage some level of continued interest in the patient from family members, ultimately the level of involvement must be a matter of choice for the family. Rehabilitation workers can play an important role in helping family members resolve some of the issues involved. Where the family members are clear that they wish to care for the relative, training should be provided, with the therapist having a continuing involvement.

THEORIES OF RECOVERY AFTER BRAIN INJURY

The mechanisms underlying the recovery of function after brain injury remain little understood. Immediately following brain trauma (primary brain damage) there is a period of alteration of consciousness (coma). The depth and duration of the coma is indicative of the extent of white matter destruction (Jennett and Teasdale, 1981). The brain's reaction to trauma can set up secondary processes (such as cerebral oedema) that lead to further damage (secondary brain damage). Resolution of these problems with appropriate medical management leads to the beginning of recovery which is marked by a return to consciousness. New research suggests that pharmacological intervention at this stage may be able to protect partially damaged neurones by making their biochemical environment more favourable. Research is, however, only at the experimental stage, and it may be many years before such treatments are available on a practical basis (Freed *et al.*, 1985; Sabel and Stein, 1986). Next there is a period in which spontaneous recovery may take place. It is during this period that PTA comes to an end, and continuous memory for events resumes. There are a number of studies that indicate that most recovery occurs in the first six months following injury after which the rate of spontaneous recovery slows considerably (Bond, 1979; Jennett and Teasdale, 1981). The process of recovery, however, is neither uniform nor linear; faculties recover at differing rates and recovery in an area can stop unexpectedly. In some areas recovery may be total and follow a very short time course; in other areas recovery may take longer and leave function impaired. For example, in the case of total amnesia there may be no trend towards recovery. The mechanisms which underlie the second stage in recovery are almost totally unknown, but continue to be the subject of speculation under the general heading of 'plasticity'. A growing number of publications attest to the great interest generated in this area (Devor, 1982; Bach-y-Rita, 1983; Illis, 1983). It is hoped that increased knowledge of the processes involved will lead to more effective rehabilitation (Bach-y-Rita, 1983; Illis, 1983). A vast number of mechanisms have been proposed, but can be grouped into two kinds of explanations of recovery of function: restitution and substitution.

RESTITUTION

1. Diaschisis

Diaschisis is the hypothesised suspension of function as a

reaction of surviving neurones to destruction of remote but connected neurones (Monakow, 1914). After an unspecified period the 'depressed' neurones recover their ability to function. Up to the end of the 1970s limited evidence was available to support the theory of diaschisis with the only well-conducted experimental test of the notion providing negative results (West et al., 1976). Recently, robust evidence for the existence of diaschisis (though not for its involvement in recovery of function) has come from studies of cerebellar blood flow in relation to space-occupying supratentorial lesions on the contralateral side. This 'crossed cerebellar diaschisis' has been reported by Baron et al. (1980) and others (Fukuyama et al., 1986; Pantano et al., 1968) and is thought to be the result of damage to descending fibres from the cerebral cortex to the cerebellum. This kind of research has only become possible with the introduction of computerised tomography (CT), nuclear magnetic resonance (NMR) and positron emission tomography (PET), which allow the possibility of much greater insight into the dynamic processes operating in a living brain. More rigorous evidence for the place of diaschisis in recovery of function after brain injury may await the application of these new techniques. Nevertheless the role of diaschisis in recovery of function after brain injury remains debatable (Schoenfeld and Hamilton, 1977; Finger and Stein, 1982). The notion of diaschisis will probably become redundant as its component processes become known.

2. Denervation supersensitivity

This theory suggests that when the number of dendrites impinging on an intact neurone is reduced it becomes more sensitive to the ones which remain (Cannon and Rosenblueth, 1949). Denervation supersensitivity has received some support (Glick and Greenstein, 1973), but the length and duration of the process is unclear. Denervation supersensitivity cannot on its own account for recovery of function since it presupposes sparing of some capacity in a given system and is therefore probably best considered in conjunction with redundancy theories discussed below (Finger and Stein, 1982). Denervation supersensitivity has also been associated with maladaptive consequences such as spasticity (Finger and Stein, 1982).

9

3. Regeneration

Functional regeneration of severed axons only occurs in the peripheral nervous system (Schoenfeld and Hamilton, 1977). To be effective a viable axon would have to reconnect to its previous target cells or to cells serving a similar function. There is little evidence for this type of connection reforming in the CNS in man. However this is an area of considerable interest since if the conditions necessary for regeneration in the CNS could become known then it may be possible to produce them by pharmacological interventions (Laurence and Stein, 1978).

4. Collateral sprouting

Collateral sprouting (or reactive synaptogenesis) concerns non-lesioned neurones which take over the site of a synaptic junction no longer occupied by the lesioned cells. Unlike regeneration there is good evidence that this process does take place in animals. Collateral sprouting may underlie some recovery of function in the CNS, but its effect is probably limited and may not always be beneficial. It has been implicated in spasticity (Liu and Chambers, 1958), and could produce 'noise' in the system by making inappropriate non-functional connections.

SUBSTITUTION

1. Redundancy and 'unmasking'

Redundancy and unmasking are theories of how the brain is organised, and make up a theory of sparing rather than of recovery. Redundancy suggests that there was in the brain, prior to injury, functional capacity which was surplus to requirements. The strongest statement of this view is the theory of equipotentiality (Tizard, 1959). According to this theory brain tissue has the capacity to subserve any function with functions distributed over the entire cortex. It is clear from the sometimes devastating deficits that can be produced by very small lesions that the theory of equipotentiality does not accord with our current knowledge (Powell, 1979). A weaker version of the theory (Pribram, 1968; Powell, 1979) views brain systems in terms of their level of redundancy. A system with high redundancy is one where the importance of an individual neurone is reduced as others may carry the same information. A system with low redundancy is one where all neurones subserve different functions so that the loss of one results in loss of the information it would have carried. As it stands this theory is not testable. There are, however, studies that suggest that recovery can be subserved by a very small percentage of surviving neurones in a system if the circumstances are favourable (Bach-y-Rita, 1980). It may be that when some — or even most — of a particular area is destroyed enough tissue remains to carry out the required behaviour in an apparently normal manner. This may in part be explained by the extreme redundancy of cues normally available in the environment and the use the CNS normally makes of this redundancy (Gibson, 1950, 1966; Barlow, 1985). Deficits may therefore only become evident with more refined testing (Laurence and Stein, 1978).

Unmasking of 'hidden' connections has also been proposed as an explanation of recovery of function. Unmasking has been defined by Bach-y-Rita (1981) as 'calling on anatomically established synapses when the usually dominating system fails'. The most notable example in man is probably the capacity for speech retained by the non-dominant hemisphere (but see below). Unfortunately what is unmasked may not improve function, and may produce an irrelevant over-determination in one system and does not subserve recovery in the damaged system.

It remains to discuss the suggestion that the brain may demonstrate more equipotentiality in early development than it does at maturity. In general terms this does seem to be the case, however, as noted by Finger and Stein (1982); the highly enthusiastic statements that were made during the 1940s and 1950s about the ability of the child's nervous system to recover from insult are rarely made today in unqualified form. Evidence from prospective studies suggests that serious brain injury produced serious consequences even at quite a young age (Heiskanen and Kaste, 1974). It has also become clear that brain-injured children who do not show immediate deficits may nevertheless do so at a later stage in their development (Milner, 1974; Bigler and Nangle, 1985).

2. Neurological substitution

This theory suggests that brain systems can change function and that the brain can relearn a lost function in an undamaged area of the brain. Miller (1985) has highlighted some of the difficulties involved in determining the possible role of neurological substitution in recovery of function. For neurological substitution to be clearly responsible for recovery of function it would be necessary to demonstrate that (1) a part of the brain not previously involved in a function becomes involved, (2) that the part of the brain subserving the role now never had the role in the past, and (3) that the function is not simply being performed by use of substitute strategies. These factors have not been adequately taken into account in most work claiming to demonstrate neurological substitution (Miller, 1985). So, for example, the right hemisphere has been shown to be active during speech production following unilateral left hemisphere damage in severely impaired non-fluent aphasics (Cummings *et al.*, 1979). There is, however, significant right hemisphere involvement in speech early in life (Hecaen and Albert, 1978) so it is more likely to be a case of unmasking than of substitution.

3. Behavioural compensation

Behavioural compensation is not a theory of neural plasticity but rather suggests that the individual, employing undamaged brain systems, adopts the use of strategies which were not used prior to injury. The use of this type of compensation has been demonstrated in animals as well as man. Rats, for example, when deprived of sight may use their sense of smell to navigate a maze. The behavioural compensation hypothesis of recovery is not a theory of plasticity because it requires no essential changes in the existing functions of undamaged brain areas. Clearly this model often involves new learning and requires the individual to accommodate to the absence of cues and to make use of new cues. Some authors regard the vast majority of cases of recovery of function as the result of employing an alternate behavioural strategy (Gazzaniga, 1978). For example a patient might be unable to translate visually presented material into language but is able to do so if he traces the outline of the image with his finger (Landis *et al.*, 1982).

There is increasing evidence that changes in the CNS take place normally as a response to changes in both the internal and external environment. For example changes in dendritic arborisation may be part of a general process in all normal adults and are not a specific response to brain injury. As Laurence and Stein (1978) point out these types of structural changes may not indicate any fundamental change in the ground rules by which the brain operates. Some authors seem to regard any form of learning (or consistent behavioural change) as evidence of neural plasticity (Bach-y-Rita, 1981). This is unhelpful since the term is then no longer reserved for *abnormal* activity in the brain which underlies recovery of function. Recovery need not imply changes in 'neural topography' if the patient employs novel tactics or unusual behaviours. The view that all recovery of function after brain injury is by definition 'plasticity' fails to examine the possible role of learning in recovery of function (Yu, 1976, 1983) or expands the meaning of the term plasticity until it becomes meaningless. It is possible that the morphological changes seen in the brain after lesion underlie recovery (Illis, 1983). However such changes may also impede recovery (Devor, 1982).

That the brain can compensate in some ways after loss of brain substance is clear. How it does so is a matter of conjecture. What is clear is that the efficacy of available techniques to assist the brain's regenerative ability is limited. Severe brain injury continues to leave patients with significant deficits. The amount of recovery possible may be related to the redundancy (spare capacity) in the brain and the way that the particular system is organised. Control of the motor system, for example, is widely distributed, involving among other areas the cerebral cortex, the basal ganglia and the cerebellum.

Currently, theories of long-term neurological recovery from brain injury offer little by way of guidance to the therapist. The most consistent suggestions from researchers into plasticity involve motivating, practical and repeated training in functional tasks (Yu, 1976; Bach-y-Rita, 1980; Finger and Stein, 1982). This type of intervention is defensible in terms that do not require recourse to theories of neural plasticity.

IS REHABILITATION EFFECTIVE?

During the period immediately following injury it is clear that energetic management by an acute trauma team can improve outcome (Becker *et al.*, 1977; Klauber *et al.*, 1985). After the acute period the role of therapeutic interventions in facilitating recovery is less clear. Studies examining the efficacy of therapeutic interventions with the brain-injured are rare. Similar influences may operate on the recovery processes on patients with cerebrovascular accidents (CVA) and those with traumatic brain injury.

The evidence for physical and for cognitive aspects of rehabilitation is discussed. A number of problems complicate the assessment of recovery after trauma to the CNS. Firstly, as noted above, patients make considerable natural recovery from brain trauma for the first six months after injury, and to a lesser degree thereafter. However the actual recovery in any individual patient is not fully predictable, making the matching of patients for controlled trials difficult. A second complication is that factors relating to recovery (particularly initial severity) may determine how much therapy a patient receives (Brocklehurst, 1978; Wade *et al.*, 1984). In regard to physical rehabilitation, three major questions have been addressed: 'Does therapy affect physical outcome?', 'When should therapy be initiated?' and 'Is one form of therapy more effective than another?'

Lind (1982) has reviewed seven studies of stroke rehabilitation, concluding that improvements attributable to rehabilitation programmes are so slight as to be unreliable. As might be expected the greatest factor in improvement was spontaneous recovery. However, Lind concludes that patients with residual functional impairments may benefit from individually tailored retraining programmes to increase independence and to prevent or reverse institutionalisation. Lind suggests that this approach could permit a substantial improvement in the quality of life for a limited number of patients (Lind, 1982).

Studies comparing types of intervention have been more straightforward. In trials which have compared the effectiveness of neurodevelopmental approaches such as those advocated by the Bobaths (Bobath, 1978), with the training of functional skills, no significant difference has been found between the two even when the neurodevelopmental treatment has involved considerably more therapy hours (Lord and Hall,

1986; Stern et al., 1970; Logigan et al., 1983).

The results of a number of studies have indicated that early intervention is preferable to later intervention (Cope and Hall, 1982; Novak et al., 1984). Novak and co-workers (1984) examined this question and found that time since injury had a small effect on response to treatment. However, they note that treatment has to be delayed by years rather than days before there is any appreciable effect. In Cope and Hall's study severely brain-injured patients in an acute rehabilitation setting were divided retrospectively into early and late rehabilitation admission groups (admitted before and after 35 days post-injury). Two groups of 16 and 20 patients were matched for length of coma, age, level of disability and neurosurgical procedures required. Findings indicated that late-admission patients required twice as much rehabilitation to reach a standard discharge criteria as did the early-admission group. Outcome at two-year follow-up was comparable. Unfortunately no reasons are given as to why the later group were not admitted to rehabilitation sooner. Since there is a range of complications which can present themselves after severe brain injury it is possible that whatever caused the delay in admission to rehabilitation services also caused the slow response to these services (Cope and Hall, 1982). Other authors have cautioned against attempting to speed recovery by including the patient prematurely in an intensive rehabilitation programme (Long et al., 1984). Shaw and co-workers (1985) describe the problems of two patients admitted and discharged from rehabilitation programmes too early. Later these patients were only 'rescued' from a nursing home setting because they were proving trouble-some to nursing staff. Provided with appropriate and timely rehabilitation both patients considerably improved their level of functioning, one patient living independently and one in a transitional living facility (Shaw et al., 1985).

Prigatano and co-workers (1984) report on the effect of a six-month intensive post-acute rehabilitation programme for severely traumatically brain-injured young adults (mean time post-injury 21.6 months). The study consisted of a comparison of 18 treated patients and 17 untreated controls. The treatment group showed a slightly greater improvement over controls on neuropsychological measures. Psychosocial adjustment was substantially improved in the treatment group versus the controls. In their discussion the authors suggest that patients most likely to benefit have an affective problem representing problems in coping with disability, and have a good work history prior to brain injury. Patients with residual impairment, but who can be taught compensatory methods, make the best candidates for rehabilitation (Prigatano *et al.*, 1984).

Evidence relating to the efficacy of cognitive and perceptual training is extremely diverse and a full review will not be attempted here. Well-designed studies that have examined the type of approach that is standard for perceptual and cognitive deficits in British and American occupational therapy departments have found them to be uniformly ineffective. A number of studies have found positive treatment effects but these studies have been poorly designed or have not taken spontaneous recovery into consideration (Lundgren and Persechino, 1986). Lincoln *et al.* (1985) compared two group approaches to perceptual disorders in a group of 33 patients with CVA and traumatic brain injury. The active treatment group received practice on 'perceptual tasks' using various types of games. The conventional therapy group did not practise tasks that were thought to improve perceptual abilities. No significant difference was found between the two groups. Since both groups improved it was suggested that this was an effect of the intensive rehabilitation programme which was present in both groups. However, time post-injury is not discussed, so it is possible that improvement was due to spontaneous recovery.

A study of a remediation programme for left-sided neglect in adult CVA patients did indicate generalisation from non-functional perceptual training to functional (ADL) skills (Diller *et al.*, 1974). A recent study by the same group of workers (Gordon *et al.*, 1985) demonstrated that the perceptual retraining of right hemisphere brain-damaged adults affected the curve of recovery but not its ultimate outcome. An attempt to replicate the findings of transfer of skills to independent ADL measures was unsuccessful. The authors suggest that attempts to rush the patient through the programme without allowing enough time for overlearning may have accounted for the disappointing results. Similarly, well-controlled trials of attempts to remediate the purely cognitive components of attention and memory have not generally demonstrated a significant treatment effect (Fussey and Tyerman, 1985). For a contrary view see Grafman (1983).

Studies that have contrasted early versus late admission to

rehabilitation programmes in the acute recovery phase in traumatically brain-injured populations have for the most part been poorly designed and inconsistent in their results (Cope and Hall, 1982; Novak *et al.*, 1984). Studies which have shown the importance of early rehabilitation may derive the effect from the avoidance of complications. Some of these issues are discussed in the next section. More consistent is the effect of post-acute rehabilitation, where there seems to be an often-repeated finding of small but significant gains where active rehabilitation is provided (Smith *et al.*, 1981; Prigatano *et al.*, 1984). This is not to argue that rehabilitation should be delayed, but does suggest that the brain-injured population can make use of rehabilitation services for considerably longer than has hitherto been thought (Long *et al.*, 1984; Shaw *et al.*, 1985).

MODELS OF THERAPY

Using 'stimulation' as a model of treatment therapists have designed hierarchical programmes designed to move the patient towards a more 'normal' level of functional performance (Rothi and Horner, 1983). This 'stimulation' model suggests that by asking the individual to perform to the limits of his ability the therapist will facilitate recovery. There are two possible arguments for this approach. The first argument best applies to the period early in recovery when it is thought that attempts to call upon a damaged system may increase changes in the brain's structure by, for example, neural regrowth. The second argument does not require changes in brain structure, and suggests that impaired functions must be maximally stimulated in order to be maintained and to develop.

As noted above, there is at present no firm evidence that neuronal regeneration underlies recovery of function. Nor is there evidence that asking a patient to perform tasks requiring cognitive skills assists neurological regeneration. Although it is generally correct to assert that practising a task improves performance (Newell and Rosenbloom, 1981) there is no evidence for a generalised effect on cognitive skills. Such a model implies the belief that cognitive skills are analogous to 'mental muscles' which become stronger with practice. As far as we are aware there is no scientific evidence that can support such a view. From a practical perspective in the early stages of recovery of function there are reasons to 'stimulate' patients which do not depend on a special theory of how to promote neural regeneration.

Patients are learning throughout the period of spontaneous recovery. Patients may learn early on that they cannot perform a task which later in the recovery process they can achieve. A patient may therefore develop a type of learned helplessness (Seligman, 1975) and have a capacity which considerably outstrips performance. If gait is taken as an example: early in treatment the patient is extremely motivated to walk, he learns a wide-based, shuffling and slow gait. Over the next few months the patient overlearns this pattern, despite the fact that he is now capable — because of improved motor coordination, posture and balance reaction — of a much more normal gait. However, only specific gait training will enable him to perform to the level of his increased capacity.

In the early part of rehabilitation one of the major roles of the therapist is to help the patient perform maximally as his condition improves. Cope (1985) describes the course of recovery of an 18-year-old man who was in a coma for nearly six months. The course of recovery was charted closely and continued for five years after the resolution of the coma. In this case the patient was provided with active rehabilitation. It is not demonstrated that the rehabilitation was causally related to the recovery, but it is realistically suggested that alternative management could have prevented the functional gains shown by this patient. Providing unnecessary assistance has been shown to reduce the independence of other institutionalised patients (Avorn and Langer, 1982) and similar considerations may apply to the brain-injured. In many senses the early rehabilitation process can be seen as an attempt to avoid complications (Rusk et al., 1969), not only the physical complications of soft tissue contractures, heterotopic ossification or decubiti, but also avoiding creating or accentuating inappropriate behaviour patterns.

The emphasis on stimulation has led to treatment approaches being adopted from which the patient is unlikely to be able to benefit. Poor memory and reduced attentional capacity indicate that if the patient is to learn, information provided must be small in amount, frequently repeated and highly motivating. Instead, therapeutic interventions have tended to be diffuse and non-specific. Therapists have used concepts such as 'judgement', 'abstraction' and 'flexibility', and where patients show deficits relating to these constructs tasks have been developed which reputedly provide practice in these 'skills'. The idea that judgement or abstraction can be practised is extremely problematic: no evidence is available to suggest that tasks used to develop them show any therapeutic effect. Many tasks used have been irrelevant to normal life outside the rehabilitation setting.

An alternative model is that of substitution (Laurence and Stein, 1978; Powell, 1981). As developed by Powell this model suggests that limited and highly directed stimulation is the key to recovery of function. The advantage of this approach is that it directs attention towards the patient's practical everyday problems. In so doing the theory avoids many of the criticisms which can be levelled against the more general 'stimulation' approach. The substitution model of treatment is based on the idea that behavioural deficits result from disorganisation of brain mechanisms rather than their loss, though both may occur. Functional skills are dependent on a large number of brain subsystems. The actual deficits in the skill performance depend on the area of the lesion and the processes involved. Therapy is aimed at providing substitute strategies within a damaged system or, when this is not possible, to encourage the development of alternative cognitive strategies. For example a therapist might attempt to facilitate the acquisition of language by the non-dominant hemisphere by translating language information into visual form (Glass *et al.*, 1973; Searleman, 1977). It is possible that some forms of carefully directed therapy might encourage this process although, as Powell (1981) has pointed out, the time period involved would probably be considerable. The effectiveness of this type of approach may depend on the type of deficit to which it is applied. For example there appears to be no neurological compensation for memory impairments which persist beyond PTA, and repeated practice of memory tasks appears to have no therapeutic advantage (Harris, 1984).

Over recent years there has been recognition of the fact that brain-injured patients can develop alternative cognitive strategies to help them overcome their cognitive deficits. Most clinicians will have seen patients who painstakingly examined objects most people would just glance at, or when given numbers to remember will group them into larger units.

Therapists have attempted to teach strategies to overcome deficits where patients have been unable to generate such compensatory strategies themselves. Some therapists have attempted to use computer programs in an effort to develop some of the impaired subskills involved in functional tasks, hoping that these will then generalise to everyday tasks that involve the skill (Young *et al.*, 1983). However the model is limited in application to the severely brain-injured for a number of reasons:

(1) *Relevance.* The skill trained must be relevant to the individual's needs and be sufficiently useful to the patient to warrant the effort needed to acquire it. A number of the internal strategies used in memory retraining do not meet this criterion. Where patients have a poor memory to start with, some of the methods may be extremely difficult to teach. Many of the techniques of imagery are limited in their usefulness to shopping lists or other highly structured situations. Some of the elaborate methods described to help patients remember faces are absurdly time-consuming with respect to the possible advantages.

(2) *Generalisation.* By generalisation we mean the ability to transfer a skill learned in one situation to other novel situations. A vast amount of evidence is available which suggests that the brain-injured have great difficulty in generalising skills (Bjoneby and Reinuang, 1985). Practice of a task leads to improvement but in the past this maxim has been taken to apply solely to perceptual-motor skills and only recently has it been recognised that it applies to learning of all kinds (Newell and Rosenbloom, 1981). Improvement in a particular task should not be taken to imply improvement in an underlying process. So for example, in regard to memory impairment, patients have improved with practice in recalling a single shopping list or in finding their way in a new environment, but this does not imply their memory has improved.

(3) *Initiation.* Brain-injured patients can often learn information but be unable to apply it. Where an individual has cognitive processing deficits in the first place compensatory techniques may not be used because they are too demanding. Patients are most likely to use techniques they have been taught if over-

learning makes them the ones requiring the least effort. Some cognitive retraining techniques are intrinsically effortful, and are as a consequence less likely to be used. It is possible to help the patient create a habit of the desired behaviour.

Rather than view the patient's deficits from the perspective of the cognitive impairments, and attempt to address these directly, it is possible to address the patient's problems from the perspective of functional skills or behavioural change. This is particularly important when a specific functional deficit impedes further progress in rehabilitation. It is often possible to train individuals in compensation habits which they have not been able to develop themselves. It is also possible to alter the environment slightly, to increase the individual's functional capacity (Gianutsos and Grynbaum, 1983).

Successful outcomes have been reported when: (a) training has addressed functional deficits, i.e. difficulty in washing and dressing is addressed directly, not the memory problem which is thought to underlie it; (b) training has been highly structured; and (c) training has been based on behavioural principles. It is therefore necessary to stress the importance of specificity and function rather than non-specific approaches.

By adopting a behavioural perspective the range of problems that can be addressed is vastly increased. Patients with severe brain injuries may display behaviour disorders which make them extremely unpopular with therapy staff. In some cases behaviour disorders may completely sabotage attempts at rehabilitation. Therapists may feel that they expend more time and energy in attempting to 'deal' with the patient's behaviour disorder than in the practice of rehabilitation, while at the same time the behaviour disorder is never directly addressed. Adopting a behavioural approach vastly expands the types of behaviours that can be addressed, and successful outcomes have been reported (Horton and Howe, 1981).

A BEHAVIOURAL APPROACH TO BRAIN INJURY REHABILITATION

A behavioural approach offers clear advantages over other available methods in brain injury rehabilitation. Learning theory offers a structure for rehabilitation with emphasis placed on measurable and reproducible techniques. Behavioural assessment and behaviour therapy look at real-life situations and state goals with clear criteria for success and failure. Brain-injured patients frequently undergo neurological and neuro-psychological tests, but there is no clear way to relate test performance to functional deficits (Bennett-Levy and Powell, 1980). Behavioural assessment (more fully described in Chapter 3) can help pinpoint how adaptive behaviours break down, examine how environmental contingencies maintain unwanted behaviours, and evaluate the functional consequences of organic damage. The form of recording may vary depending on level of impairment and areas of deficit, but the most important is naturalistic, leading to structured observation which records antecedent, behaviour and consequence (ABC). Observation needs to cover a wide range of behavioural settings and levels of stress on the patient. Areas examined may include social interaction, self-care, leisure and family interaction. Some extremely significant behaviour disorders may only become evident in response to a very limited range of cues. For example aggressive behaviour might only be displayed with family members after drinking alcohol. A behavioural approach helps in the selection of appropriate goals and in assessing the patient's response to treatment. The discipline of establishing a baseline, designing an intervention strategy and operationally assessing the patient response to treatment helps clinicians avoid such vague goals as 'develop abstraction'. Behavioural techniques cover a wide range of possible strategies and are problem-orientated.

Conditioning methods may not at first sight seem appropriate for use with the brain-injured since these patients are likely to have problems with new learning. However it is widely recog-nised that other groups who have impaired learning ability have benefited from behavioural methodology. For example many regard behaviour therapy as fundamental to the training of the mentally handicapped. Even profoundly retarded individuals can learn complex tasks when training is adapted to their needs. A number of studies have demonstrated the similar learning characteristics of the mentally handicapped and the brain-injured (Miller, 1980; Wood, 1986b). Among the most significant methods of learning in this group are

(1) *Associative learning.* Both classical (Pavlov, 1927) and

operant (Skinner, 1938) learning are concerned with the causal relationships between events in the organism's environment. This type of learning is thought to be mediated by subcortical brain structures and can be contrasted with:

(2) *Cognitive learning.* This involves the formation of representations (often linguistic in man) which are apparently dependent on the neocortex and hippocampus to establish rules and regularities about the environment (Goldstein and Oakley, 1985). Both memory and attentional deficits can hamper the severely brain-injured individual's ability to benefit from cognitive learning. However, by repeatedly presenting the information the individual needs to acquire in exactly the same way, and by making this process rewarding, the individual's chances of learning can be maximised.

A complex interaction of many types of learning is probably present in the acquisition of most types of learned behaviour in man. Although the specifics of an intervention will depend on the type of learning thought to predominate, in general terms behavioural techniques aid in the mapping of relationships between events occurring in the environment (Mackintosh, 1983). The key to this is reinforcement, being an event following a behaviour which increases the rate of recurrence of the behaviour.

The state of the damaged brain is of fundamental importance in assessing how to best facilitate learning in the patient. Powell (1981) has emphasised the importance of considering the triad of behaviour, cognition and neurophysiology. From a behavioural perspective this view represents a retreat from the 'black box' view of behaviour in which accounts of internal factors in learning would be eschewed as mentalistic. This is a return to the views of Hull (1952) where an 'O' for organism is incorporated into the S–R chain (S–O–R). Attempts can be made to modify the internal environment (Chapter 2) just as the external environment can be adapted.

In examining the capacity of the injured brain for learning new or more adaptive behaviour two types of limitation have to be borne in mind. These may be labelled neuropsychiatric and neuropsychological. The first of these involves organic disorders arising from the brain injury. The second refers to static limitations to learning arising from brain injury. Neuropsychiatric disorders are not directly under the control of the individual and may often be treated medically. Examples include disorders of arousal (which at its extremes prevents most forms of purposive behaviour), epilepsy and schizophrenic or depressive-like illnesses. Disinhibition, loss of emotional control and the failure to obey social rules are associated with impairments of frontal lobe function. Patients may be hyper-sexual, be overly friendly, make gross errors of judgement and in severe cases may be completely oblivious to acceptable rules of social behaviour (to the extent that some patients will fondle total strangers or masturbate or defaecate in public). Lishman and others (Lishman, 1978; Elisinger and Damasio, 1984) have underlined that such changes may occur independently of pre-morbid behaviour. So-called 'limbic epilepsy' or temporal lobe epilepsy has been implicated in a range of bizarre behaviours and aggressive outbursts (Blumer, 1970; Hoshmand and Brawley, 1970; Bear, 1983). This is not to suggest, however, that environmental manipulation is inappropriate in helping patients in these circumstances. Wood (1986a) has demonstrated that some patients are unable to benefit from either behavioural or pharmacological approaches, but are able to benefit when these were used in combination. Similar drug/behaviour therapy interactions have been demonstrated in other patient popula-tions (Rappaport et al., 1983).

It is also reasonable to consider in the category of organic disorders lack of insight, obsessionality and paranoid ideas, as well as some of the more well-known organic conditions such as the symptom complex which has been likened to the Kluver–Bucy syndrome in monkeys, and which is characterised by visual agnosia, oral tendencies, hyperactivity, placidity and hypersexuality. Careful evaluation by an experienced specialist is essential, as some of these disorders can present as apparently pure behaviour disorders; temporal lobe epilepsy as aggressive outbursts or a depressive illness as poor motivation. Alterna-tively behavioural deficits can be misdiagnosed as psychiatric illness (Shaw et al., 1985).

Within the category of neuropsychological disorders are impairments in the learning processes themselves. Underlying these may be a range of perceptual deficits, impaired memory, attention or motivation. Reduced attentional and informational processing capacity may in themselves play a part in producing bizarre behaviours since the patient does not respond to available situational cues. Oakley (Oakley, 1983; Goldstein and Oakley, 1985) has related a number of studies with experimentally brain-damaged animals to rehabilitation with the traumatically brain-injured. Human and animal studies are used to illustrate that associative learning may remain intact after brain injury, possibly due to its being dependent on subcortical brain structures. Goldstein and Oakley (1985) suggest that application of associational learning based on behaviour modification techniques may lead to the development of adequate behavioural control, thus allowing the use of cognitive therapies. The same authors underline the importance of attentional variables in learning in both animals and man (Goldstein and Oakley, 1985). There are two related problems in the application of behavioural methods in this group: the time needed for conditioning to take place and the frequency of reinforcement necessary to achieve it (Wood and Eames, 1981). The process of learning in the brain-injured is often protracted.

Impaired memory does appear to play a part in this slowed learning process. However, it does not seem to account for all of the differences as two patients with amnesic syndromes who respond in similar ways to psychological testing may learn at very different rates. Attentional deficits and differing learning methods may account for some of the differences. Many patients are so badly damaged that they pay little attention to their environment. Indeed some degree of attentional deficit has been noted to be one of the most frequent consequences of brain injury (Van Zomeren and Deelman, 1978; Gronwall and Wrightson, 1981). If patients do not attend to regularities in their environment they may have more difficulty learning from them. By pairing the naturally occurring environmental consequences with additional consequences it is possible to make the effects of a particular behaviour more salient to the patient. Reinforcement assists learning in normal, retarded, and brain-injured populations (Ellis, 1970; Lashley and Drabman, 1974; Dolan and Norton, 1977). The importance of tangible reinforcement in addition to social praise is less clear, and results have been inconsistent (Lashley and Drabman, 1974; Dolan and Norton, 1977; Dolan, 1979). Dolan has suggested that the inconsistency may result from the level of motivation towards what is to be taught: where the subject is highly motivated tangible rewards may be irrelevant. This view accords with our own clinical impressions. Many brain-injured patients are under-motivated or motivated towards unrealistic or inappropriate ends. Behavioural techniques, while not solving the problem, can help therapists manipulate the environment to help overcome motivational problems.

The problems behaviour modification can address in the brain-injured population can be divided into three types (Eames and Wood, 1985a): positive behaviour disorder, negative behaviour disorder and specific skill deficit. Behavioural interventions attempt to modify established automatic behaviour patterns by manipulating reinforcement.

Stern and his co-workers have examined behaviour disturbance as a function of severity of cerebral damage. The authors attempted to examine four areas of symptomatology: behaviour, personality, affect and cognition. The authors do not establish the separate identities of these symptom complexes but their research does indicate that the more severe the diffuse injury the less behaviour the individual is likely to produce. Their results suggest a complex interrelation between disinhibition, ability to initiate behaviour and arousal in determining positive and negative behaviour disorder. With extremely severe damage the degree of disinhibition may be masked by a generalised paucity of behaviour described by Lishman (1978) as slowing, inertia and aspontaneity. In an analysis of personality and behavioural change after severe blunt head injury Brooks and McKinlay (1983) found that most patients were rated as showing increased temper and irritability and decreased energy and enthusiasm. The authors suggest that these changes are a very common consequence of severe brain injury (Brooks and McKinlay, 1983). Our clinical impression is that the more severe the diffuse injury the more the individual has difficulty in initiating behaviour.

Specific skill deficits include mobility, washing, dressing, continence and navigation. Not only does a behavioural approach provide opportunities to manipulate motivational factors, but breaking down tasks into component steps appears to help patients learn. It enables the behaviour to be understood more easily by the patient and to be replicated, allowing for consistent practice.

As yet very little work attempts to relate site of lesion with response to behavioural techniques. No predictor of behavioural learning has been reported, though the work of Miller (1980) represents a useful beginning. Petrides (1985) has, however, reported a study which suggests that patients with damage to parts of the frontal cortex may have problems with conditional associative learning tasks. Behavioural learning with the patient with memory impairment (which may imply damage to specific brain structures) is not only possible but definitely indicated in the development of both behavioural control and specific skill development (Glisky *et al.*, 1986).

Eames and Wood (1985b) have described a unit for the treatment of the severely brain-injured run as a token economy for patients whose disturbed behaviours prevented them from benefiting from therapy aimed at reducing their physical, behavioural and functional skills deficits. The methods used are similar to those used in the management of severe behaviour disorders in other populations, but have not hitherto been used with this population (Kazdin and Bootzin, 1972; Wood, 1984).

The behavioural treatment is based on positive reinforcement of appropriate behaviours (social reinforcement, attention and praise plus tangible reinforcement, e.g. chocolate, soft drinks, cigarettes or other privileges). In order not to support inappropriate behaviour by social interaction a 'time-out on the spot' (TOOTS) procedure is used. TOOTS is an extinction method based on removing from the subject the opportunity of gaining positive reinforcement contingent upon the subject producing an unwanted behaviour, and is adapted from the behavioural procedure of time-out (Ullmann and Krasner, 1969). Episodes of physical aggression led to a time-out for 5 minutes in a time-out room. These methods are more fully described elsewhere (Eames and Wood, 1985b). Within this context patients are taught positive behaviour and skills to increase their performance and quality of life.

A recent follow-up study examined a consecutive series of 24 patients treated on this unit. Time since discharge ranged from 6 to 39 months with a mean of 18.8 months. The principal outcome measure used was a hierarchical scale of placements ranked in terms of quality of life for the patient (Eames and Wood, 1985b). The results of the study show improvement in behaviour and subsequent placement. There was no trend towards relapse as time from discharge increased, nor was length of time since treatment a factor which reduced response to treatment.

Mean interval between injury and admission to the unit was four years, and the condition of all patients on admission was considered static in that it was highly unlikely that they would make further improvement. Most available outcome studies do not mention treatment (Jennett and Teasdale, 1981). This report suggests that even years after injury highly structured, directed and persistent rehabilitation can achieve changes significant enough to make valuable improvements in quality of life. In practice length of stay in this kind of programme needs to be considerable. Although this kind of intervention is costly it would appear justified if it leads to greater independence from long periods of unnecessary institutional care.

Despite the efficacy of these types of techniques with this patient population behavioural methods have been remarkably under-utilised, as evidenced by the small number of reports specifically advocating its use with the traumatically brain-injured (Horton and Howe, 1981; Eames and Wood, 1985a,b). Recently, however, a number of workers have recommended its use on theoretical grounds (Goldstein and Oakley, 1985; Oakley, 1983; Miller, 1980).

Post-acute rehabilitation of the brain-injured is the exception rather than the rule. Most rehabilitation programmes are conducted when patients are still in the period of spontaneous recovery, with treatment being terminated when the patient ceases to 'make progress' (Gilchrist and Wilkinson, 1979). Unfortunately it is precisely at this time that lasting deficits are becoming apparent. Some staff may dislike using behavioural methods, believing them to be demeaning to the patient. As with any treatment, guidelines should govern its application. However, patients have a right to adequate and appropriate treatment. Often patients are unable to make use of less structured approaches and may suffer considerably in terms of quality of life and future placement if behaviour disorders or skills deficits are not ameliorated. Individuals who object to the use of behavioural interventions on philosophical grounds need to demonstrate that there are alternatives which can produce the improvements in the patient's quality of life provided by behavioural methodologies.

SUMMARY

Following severe brain injury most patients have cognitive deficits which are likely to interfere with their ability to make use of standard rehabilitation approaches. After the initial stages of recovery patients are often left with cognitive, behavioural and physical deficits. The more severe the deficits the more likely the individual is to be dependent, often putting great stress on family or care staff. Patients are left in highly inappropriate settings, exacerbating the management problems and often causing deterioration in self-help skills and social behaviour. Behavioural learning programmes are particularly flexible in meeting the patient's needs, and can be used to present information in a way which maximises the individual's chances for learning. The fact that even very handicapped patients have retained some capacity for new learning means that it is possible to teach patients new skills which increase their independence and reduce their unacceptable behaviour.

2

Medical Considerations in Brain Injury Rehabilitation

Martyn Rose

INTRODUCTION

Brain injury does not affect a representative cross-section of the population. The group is to some extent self-selecting with young 'extrovert' males predominating. The rehabilitation team needs to be aware of this as they try to draw out 'normal' function and behaviour from their patient group.

The brain-damaged adult has different management requirements at each stage of recovery. In the early stages supportive and preventive measures assume primary importance. Subsequently re-education (as supplied by 'physical' therapists) is needed, whilst later still there is need for a combination of support (but no more than is necessary) and replacement or substitution for the abilities that have been totally lost. Physical, cognitive, psychiatric, behavioural or social problems may exist in varying combination and degree. It is the neuropsychological and neuropsychiatric sequelae that produce the greatest handicap. Severity of injury can be judged by length of coma, post-traumatic amnesia, Glasgow Coma Scale score (Jennett et al., 1981) or length of time in hospital. However, there is little useful correlation between severity of injury and outcome, although combining information presumed to reflect severity can increase predictive ability (Klonoff et al., 1986). Significant numbers of people with mild-to-moderate injury continue to show symptoms attributable to the injury more than two years afterwards, whether or not there is litigation involved. The majority of those with severe injury are reported to make a 'good' recovery. For those with severe injury the recovery process appears to extend over years rather than months, and the supposition that the earlier 'active' therapy starts the better may not be entirely true. (This presupposes that 'passive' management will at least be preventing the development of problems in posture or behaviour.)

Rehabilitation facilities, demanding highly trained and motivated staff, are in lamentably short supply or non-existent, depending on the area of the country. There are discussions about plans to develop a service to the brain-injured taking place in many parts of the UK, but the reality is that NHS facilities within the UK are *contracting*. In the US services may or may not be available, depending on the state, but truly adequate care is available only to those with private health insurance. There is little evidence to show that rehabilitation works, although this is mainly because of the difficulties in carrying out adequate research in this area (*Lancet*, 1982; Eames and Wood, 1985a). Long-term management is commonly provided on an *ad hoc* basis and leaves much to be desired, especially in those cases with the greatest need. Many of the most severely handicapped people still face the prospect of placement — long-term or short-term — in hospitals for the mentally subnormal or psychogeriatric population.

MECHANISMS OF INJURY

Most brain injuries are acquired as a result of an acceleration/deceleration injury (road traffic accident (RTA) or fall). Rotational forces acting upon the brain are also generated, and the result is diffuse axonal damage (DAD). There is usually contusion to frontal and temporal poles, and to brainstem pathways and centres, whatever the site of impact. Secondary damage follows if the complications of raised intracranial pressure (RICP) and hypoxia/anoxia occur. If the injury involves skull fracture then infection can produce further problems, although the problems of RICP may then be reduced. Injury involving skull fracture looks more frightening and serious but may be associated with good outcome. Focal damage may be produced by, for example, a blow with a blunt instrument. The prognosis in such cases is usually quite good. Diffuse damage can be produced by infection, as in herpes simplex encephalitis, or anoxia after cardiac arrest. Anoxic damage carries the worst prognosis with major cognitive loss and handicapping behavioural changes. However, some people with inequivocal primary anoxic damage have no detectable cognitive loss despite major physical impairment. It will therefore be seen that the prognosis can vary dramatically from case to case. This is usually dependent upon the underlying cause of the damage, but each person should be assessed individually without preconception.

NATURAL HISTORY OF RECOVERY

Once the life-threatening situations have been controlled progressive recovery is the commonest pattern. Improvement is often seen to proceed at a variable rate with a tendency to slow down as time passes. Recovery may be in a series of steps with periods of unpredictable length in between. No one can predict rate or degree of recovery. After some time has elapsed the past rate of recovery may give some clues to the future rate, but caution in giving prognosis, and a readiness to admit ignorance, is the best policy.

An exception may be severe communication impairment, especially when deeper dominant hemisphere structures are involved. Whilst early improvement may be apparent, and 'flashes' of 'normal' communication seen, improvement may cease within only a few months. Once again it is necessary to point out, however, that prediction is not yet possible, and it must remain reasonable to strive to obtain greater function for some considerable time. Improvement in other functions has clearly been observed to continue for many years after injury with and without therapy, although late complications such as hydrocephalus may slow, stop or reverse improvement, and themselves need treatment.

The great majority of traumatically brain-injured people make good physical recovery, whilst large numbers are left with varying degrees of neuropsychological, neuropsychiatric and subsequent behavioural impairment. The effects of age on recovery are unclear. It has long been assumed that youth protects to a variable and unpredictable extent. This may not be true beyond the age of nine or ten years. Whether the prognosis for the over-60s is even worse remains to be clarified. It is essential to remember, however, that the prognosis is commonly better than most 'experts' allow.

There is no suggestion that life expectancy is reduced for any but the most dependent group, although the quality of care provided is vital for many patients. A proportion of those with partial recovery (and the retention of the ability to understand their loss) commit suicide. They may not communicate their distress or intentions clearly in advance, and vigilance on the part of carers is the most important preventive measure. Grief affects a majority of the injured and the grieving process is lengthy — certainly taking years rather than months. The grieving process is complex and may be further complicated by the need to mourn lost relationships as well as physical and 'mental' loss.

Post-traumatic epilepsy affects a proportion of brain-injured patients and the control of seizures can be difficult. For most of the brain-injured group, in the absence of risk-increasing factors, the chance of developing seizures is hardly increased and the taking of anticonvulsants is unnecessary.

Post-traumatic migraine is relatively common, possibly more so in those with better overall outcome. It is sometimes not diagnosed or treated. Prophylaxis with propranolol is often effective. There is some evidence that this problem may spontaneously resolve over two to three years and some children may lose the symptom at puberty, although some people continue to be troubled for years. Previously existing migraine has been recorded to be 'cured' by head injury.

MECHANISMS OF RECOVERY

Initially recovery follows the resolution of brain swelling, hypoxia, electrolyte imbalance and possibly neurotransmitter depletion. Recovery may be associated with axonal regrowth, collateral sprouting and the addition of neurones. Other mechanisms which may account for the restoration of function in large tracts of neurones include substitution, compensation, redundancy, interhemispheric transfer and restitution (Robinson, 1986), although see Chapter 1 for a fuller discussion.

ORGANISATION OF SERVICES

Patients and their families benefit from the care and advice of experts at every stage of the treatment and recovery process. This is true whether the injury is mild, moderate or severe. The ideal brain trauma service would provide appropriate care for all, deploying staff with a range of abilities to the patient group when needed. The patients' needs range from the management of life-threatening situations through to physical and mental well-being; from total dependence to total independence.

Rehabilitation, which is a continuous process, aims at reducing dependence to the lowest levels possible and maximising function. The services to be provided should be based on three main levels of recovery, irrespective of time from injury: early, intermediate and late. The requirements at each stage are very different and need staff of differing training and ability. The brain-damaged person has lost far more function than any other traumatised patient, whether or not there is multiple injury. Initially the 'medical model' of care is necessary, if not essential. Treatment is made more difficult not least because of the inevitable interference with learning and memory.

GENERAL PRINCIPLES OF MANAGEMENT

Rest has long been recognised as an important aspect of the management of all disease and trauma. Cerebral trauma is no exception. It is impossible to totally rest the brain but restriction of activity is important.

The *early* level of recovery is characterised by supportive, preventative and protective management. The management of the unconscious patient is well described in other texts and will not be detailed here (Jennett and Teasdale, 1981). Respiration is controlled to ensure optimal levels of oxygen and carbon dioxide and to allow some control of intracranial pressure. Steroids are increasingly thought to be of little value in the control of brain swelling after head injury, and there is no indication for prophylactic antibiotics or anticonvulsants. If anticonvulsants are required (and they may presently be over-prescribed) it is preferable to use carbamazepine if tolerated. When first prescribed it can produce drowsiness which usually diminishes to an acceptable level within five to seven days. Ataxia can be produced or worsened and may restrict use of the drug. A small proportion of people (about 3 per cent) develop a rash which invariably restricts the use of the drug. Phenytoin remains the most commonly prescribed drug despite its well-recognised adverse effects on learning and behaviour. Carbamazepine is as effective an anticonvulsant and lacks these unwanted effects (Bremer *et al.*, 1980; Hawkins *et al.*, 1985; McQueen *et al.*, 1983; Jennett *et al.*, 1973).

The background environment in which the person is nursed should be simple and uncluttered, with good lighting and a minimum of staff and visitors passing through. This approach ensures that stimuli reaching the brain-damaged patient are minimised and controlled to some extent.

Regular and careful observation of recovery of function needs to be made, to avoid the possibility of, for example, patients with well-recovered swallowing reflexes receiving continuous nasogastric feeds. There can be no reasonable indication for this to occur, bearing in mind the long-term complications such as oesophageal stenosis or chest infection. Feeding via a gastrostomy is preferable if oral intake cannot be maintained at adequate levels. Nasogastric tube feeding is necessary at first, but efforts to establish swallowing and 'normal' movements of lips, tongue and palate should be started early with the help of a speech therapist using techniques of icing and other stimulatory methods.

In the early stages even simple and essential nursing procedures such as turning the patient produce significant rises in intracranial pressure (ICP). The effect of these rises can be assumed to be potentially damaging to the recovering but vulnerable brain, and should urge caution to those who believe in 'maximal stimulation' of even comatose patients. The effect of other forms of stimulation (especially sound but also touch) is minimal, and as to whether there is any link between early stimulation and outcome remains a matter of faith amongst practitioners.

Bearing in mind the problems of impaired concentration and ready fatiguability experienced by individuals later in their recovery, if it is considered reasonable to start to commence stimulation (despite the lack of evidence as to its efficacy) it is better to use stimuli that are clear, familiar and given in short sequences with rest in between. The timing of the introduction of 'therapeutic' stimuli remains empirical. However, as there is evidence for depletion of neurotransmitter substances in the early stages of recovery this alone argues for the restriction of cerebral activity.

Chest physiotherapy is vital to ensure an adequate airway, but the effect on intracranial pressure must be remembered and therapy used accordingly. It is important to attend to the positioning of limbs to minimise spasticity and reduce the likelihood of, for example, subluxation of a paralysed shoulder.

At the *intermediate* level of recovery, supportive management continues whilst more active measures to enhance recovery are implemented.

The significantly brain-damaged person presents special challenges to therapists (including nurses), with the combination of problems which is unique to this group. Difficulties with attention, concentration, sensation, perception, information processing, learning and memory, together with the well-recognised and common loss of drive, combine to make re-learning a long, slow and tedious task for patient and therapists. It is not only the patient who must be patient.

Team treatment

Treatment is now best provided by the interdisciplinary team with the doctor as one member. In the UK the medical model of treatment (entirely necessary in the life-threatening early stages) persists throughout the period of rehabilitation, however long it may be. Thus the doctor heads the rehabilitation team. This obtains whether or not he or she has the most knowledge, interest, understanding or time; and reflects, among other things, the expectations of doctors, nurses, patients, relatives and many therapists. This system works best when the doctor recognises the therapeutic limitations of medicine (and medicines), and uses their position to provide a relatively dispassionate overview of each case. If the doctor becomes 'involved' with patient or relatives (an essential step if he is actually to treat) there is likely to be a need for someone else outside the treating team to try to set limits to treatment. This is a most difficult task, and treatment is often given for too short a time.

Treatment may be best delivered in one-to-one situations, but it is probable that combined therapy (true interdisciplinary involvement) properly applied will enhance outcome.

Behaviour

Behaviour can be a problem, with disorientation and disinhibition producing major difficulties in rehabilitation. Sedative drugs are often prescribed, but the better solution is to provide a more suitable environment with appropriate behavioural management. There is little doubt that the use of drugs in these situations is based on the needs of other patients and staff, and can be deleterious to the brain-damaged patient. Such drugs work by altering neurochemical transmission in a variety of ways. It is certain that the psychoactive drugs in use will have some unwanted effects. Habituation occurs and the dose needs to be progressively increased. Drugs may be continued when no longer required.

Researchers are presently investigating the use of low-dose haloperidol (a neuroleptic or 'major tranquilliser' which acts on dopaminergic transmission) as a suitable sedative drug. It is unfortunate that extra-pyramidal symptoms are common with this medication. In children it is said that droperidol (similar to haloperidol but with a shorter half-life) adversely affects intracranial pressure. If this is true at all stages of recovery, and is also seen in adults, then the drug should not be used. Pimozide, another type of neuroleptic, may be a more acceptable alternative but remains to be assessed. Benzodiazepines (e.g. diazepam) which modify GABA (gamma-aminobutyric acid) activity have a wide range of unwanted effects and may 'release' aggressive behaviour. They are best avoided. This may also apply to clobazam which is used as an anticonvulsant. Diazepam remains of value in the emergency control of seizures (Holland and Whalley, 1981).

Mobility

Physiotherapy continues, now aiming to promote control of position and posture whilst continuing to minimise spasticity and tremor if present. A number of types of tremor can be seen after brain injury. (In fact any symptom which can arise as a result of brain dysfunction can be seen after head/brain injury whether one considers physical or mental symptoms.) A 'bilateral' approach to improving function is most commonly adopted and is probably best even when patients fail to continue to use it. However eclecticism is wise given the total lack of evidence for any method of management. Claims have been made for the value of *electro-acupuncture* in the management of spasticity (and pain). It may be of use when there is pain, but its effect on painless spasticity is more often unremarkable. In this and other treatment areas there is room for more controlled observations.

Drugs for the control of spasticity are often tried. With the exception of dantrolene they act principally on the central nervous system. They rarely help in brain-injured people, but once started they are commonly continued. Unwanted effects include behavioural disturbance and the indications for their use after brain trauma are few. Some doctors recommend the abolition of troublesome spasticity by intramuscular injection of alcohol or phenol into motor points. Whilst there may be the occasional indication for such management it is difficult to justify the treatment of major organic disorder by the deliberate creation of further damage in areas which are not themselves the site of dysfunction. Tremor may be reduced with drugs, but there is little to be lost by waiting to see what time alone can achieve. Some tremors (especially of the basal ganglia type) may appear during recovery months after injury.

Cognitive function

Neuropsychological assessment may now add important information about problems of higher cerebral function. This specialised form of assessment (not an estimate of IQ) can discern problems of attention, concentration, perception, praxis and speed of information processing, and can make valuable contributions to treatment programmes.

Nursing

The patient's need for physical nursing (i.e. having things done for or to him) lessens as time passes. It is here that the basic skills of the nurse trained in psychiatry can be effectively applied. The psychiatric nurse has learnt how to support, encourage and motivate the most difficult of individuals and these skills are precisely those needed by the recovering patient.

The *late* phase of recovery involves retraining, provision of orthoses and environmental support.

Natural recovery may continue for an apparently indefinite

period. This may be discomfiting for those who need clear models of recovery, but most people who have worked for a number of years in the specialty will have examples of individuals who improve functionally from year to year. Impressive (if strictly limited) outcome to rehabilitation is possible even after many years, and in the most profoundly damaged people (Eames and Wood, 1985a). It has also confirmed the need for highly motivated, open-minded staff with high staff–patient ratios and lengthy treatment periods. It is clear that referral for intensive rehabilitation can be made too early when injury is profound and damage is extensive. How far this observation applies to less severely damaged people is uncertain, but those with damage concentrated in the brainstem certainly appear to make later recovery than others.

Medical assessment

It is always worth carrying out a full assessment, checking and querying all previous findings. On rare occasions serious errors of diagnosis (or at least opinion) will come to light which, on review, will profoundly alter the prognosis and management. Expert medical opinion should be sought where appropriate (orthopaedic, ophthalmic, ENT or psychiatric) and opinions discussed.

Physical and mental state need review. In particular, evidence of hypothalamic or pituitary axis dysfunction should be sought, and the need for replacement therapy assessed. Drug therapy must be reviewed and the possibility of reductions in dosage considered. There are occasions when drugs, previously prescribed on an apparently empirical basis, have so unequivocally enhanced function that they should be continued or at most discontinued on a well-controlled trial basis. Anticonvulsants may not be necessary, but the individual's need for antidepressants should be assessed. At this assessment the doctor must also consider the place of surgery, especially for fixed deformity at any joint. Heterotopic ossification may be evident and treatment indicated. It is rarely easy to recommend an 'aggressive' (usually surgical) approach in the profoundly damaged person but everyone has the right for reasonable treatment approaches to be considered, and 'safe' but less than adequate management may be regretted later.

In some cases with severe (basal ganglia type) tremor thalamotomy may be considered. Personal experience recalls two cases. Both underwent unilateral thalamotomy after appropriate assessment and both had significant reduction of tremor. However, functionally and behaviourally both showed significant loss, and on subsequent review there is no doubt that in terms of tremor one patient was worse off after operation and the other unhelped. Consideration may be given to cerebellar electrode implants and chronic stimulation, mainly to treat severe spasticity, although beneficial effects on behaviour have been reported. Unfortunately the operation is not readily available. As the technique employs stimulation and not ablation it is hoped that adverse effects will be non-existent or minimal. In general the use of any technique is not recommended in which more nervous tissue will be damaged or destroyed.

NEUROPSYCHIATRIC ASSESSMENT

Abormalities of mental state are common after traumatic brain injury (Feigenson *et al.*, 1977; Storey, 1970). Some are particularly difficult to diagnose. Psychiatric diagnosis relies mainly on the correct interpretation of verbally obtained material usually gathered at semi-structured interview. Observation of sleep pattern, physical concomitants of anxiety or behaviour patterns may arouse enough suspicion of psychiatric disease to justify a trial of treatment. In difficult cases it is usually reasonable to risk treatment of a possibly non-existent disease rather than to fail to treat one which is present and limiting response to other treatment.

Depressive illness can be particularly hard to detect but sleep disturbance (early morning wakening and/or difficulty getting to sleep), impaired appetite and loss of interest should alert carers to this possibility. A trial of antidepressant medication will usually enable the diagnosis to be confirmed or refuted with confidence. It is important, however to remember the unwanted effects of most antidepressants, such as sedation, dryness of mouth, impaired vision, cardiotoxicity and precipitation of epilepsy. Clearly these drugs are to be used in *illness* and not solely because of 'unhappiness'. There may, of course, be a continuum from simple unhappiness through to severe depressive illness, but clinical judgement will have to be exercised in deciding on treatment. However, Schmidt (1969) found that depression was an important prognostic factor in response to rehabilitation.

Mania does occur, and is usually easier to diagnose. It should not be confused with euphoria. The response to treatment is often better than that of depression. Lithium may be indicated even when its side-effect of tremor causes a worsening control of movement.

Obsessionality and ritualistic behaviour are becoming more widely recognised as complications of brain injury arising *de novo*. Management is often difficult and in severe cases is unsuccessful. Neither drug therapy (clomipramine has been recommended) nor behavioural therapy has been shown to be effective. This particular symptom, resulting as it can do in the hoarding of goods, may make the individual unacceptable in a number of long-term placements.

Dissociative (hysterical) behaviour may appear in people without a pre-existing hysterical personal trait. A strict behavioural approach to rehabilitation has not helped such individuals (who appear indifferent to reward or even 'punishment') and may have been instrumental in producing deterioration in some people. A less demanding approach — allowing the individual more 'choice' — but still containing elements of environmental control, is often more effective. In broad terms, however, the appearance of 'negative' or 'opposite' behaviours (i.e. the person does the opposite of what is asked, thereby implying understanding of the command or request) should warn the rehabilitation team of considerable difficulties ahead.

Schizophreniform or psychotic illnesses of various types are seen in a small number of brain-injured patients. Diagnosis can be particularly difficult and a trial of neuroleptic medication may be required. Pimozide can be valuable in cases of 'overactivity', and propranolol in high dosage may be effective with overactivity/overarousal and sometimes aggression. (The latter drug cannot be used in people with asthma, and on occasions may precipitate hallucinations and bizarre behaviour.)

Other problems

Vasopressin may have effects on arousal/attention and memory as well as relieving diabetes insipidus (although at differing doses). The evidence for the efficacy of this naturally occurring brain hormone is uncertain, and studies to evaluate its worth continue. At the present state of knowledge a trial of lypressin nasal spray (one squirt into each nostril twice in the day for one month) should be considered for individuals with problems of arousal/attention and consequent memory difficulty.

SUMMARY

Head trauma occurs in a group which is to some extent self-selecting and is predominantly young, previously physically healthy and male. Significant problems after the earliest stages are mainly to be found in the neuropsychological and neuro-psychiatric fields. Management should aim to match the individual to his environment. At present the use of drugs is empirical, often unnecessary and potentially or actually harmful.

Whilst improvements can be expected to take place in early diagnosis and management it is essential for improvements to be made in the longer-term care — in both rehabilitation and long-term placement facilities.

3

The Psychological Management of Behaviour Disorders Following Brian Injury

Rodger Ll. Wood and Paul W. Burgess

INTRODUCTION

The studies by Brooks and his colleagues in Glasgow have highlighted the importance of brain-injured patients being able to display appropriate social behaviour in order for them to be accepted back into the community (Brooks and McKinlay, 1983; Brooks, 1984). Brain injury rehabilitation is beginning to give proper attention to disorders of behaviour, because inappropriate behaviour can make it difficult for therapists to provide patients with the right quality or quantity of rehabilitation, thereby directly affecting their potential for recovery (Fordyce *et al.*, 1985).

Methods for dealing with different types of behaviour disorders have been presented by Wood and Eames (1981) and Wood (1984, 1987). These clinical examples suggest that a variety of behaviour management techniques are needed to deal with different types of unacceptable behaviour. This chapter reviews those behaviour management techniques that have developed from clinical psychology and are now being applied in the management of the neurobehaviourally disturbed patient. Consideration is given to how these techniques may best be administered in the setting of a brain injury rehabilitation unit, in order to control and eliminate disorders of behaviour, while promoting the development of independence in social and functional skills.

TYPES OF ORGANICALLY DETERMINED BEHAVIOUR DISORDER

Behaviour disorders which emerge during recovery from brain

43

injury can be considered from several perspectives. One broad distinction is to separate psychological reactions *to* injury from behaviour responses which are a direct consequence *of* the injury. This is an important distinction because it identifies some behaviours as being neurologically or organically generated and therefore not under (or minimally under) the control of the individual. Other behaviours, however, can be regarded either as more purposeful, or motivated by some emotional reaction, or as a consequence of the psychological disposition of an individual who is distressed by the change of status and level of independence which commonly occurs following brain injury.

Once this major division between a psychological reaction and neurologically mediated behaviour has been made it becomes necessary to consider different types of abnormalities within those two broad categories. Wood and Eames (1981) and Wood (1987) describe how some aggressive responses are evinced as a direct consequence of abnormal electrical activity while other forms of aggression are due to damaged inhibitory or modulatory mechanisms which normally control our response to frustration. After severe brain injury, electrical abnormalities may be combined with loss of inhibitory controls, producing serious aggressive disorders. These will not respond to psychological methods of management alone, and need to be regulated by appropriate anticonvulsants to help stabilise mood and reduce impulsivity.

Aggressive responses which have an organic basis often possess a different quality from psychologically based aggressive reactions, and they may also occur more frequently. Aggressive behaviour that has psychological origins may be predicted from its pattern of occurrence, which has some purposeful or goal-directed quality. Organically mediated aggression, on the other hand, is often characterised by a lack of any apparent pattern or display of gratification on the part of the individual who exhibits that aggression. Indeed, it is often the case that following an aggressive outburst, patients who have an organic aetiology for their disorder will apologise profusely and show considerable remorse. In contrast, behaviour which is psychologically generated is usually not associated with any contrite attitude on the part of the patient. This type of aggression can often be associated with attention-seeking behaviour which uses an aggressive response as a means to an end.

Perhaps the next major distinction between behaviour disorders should be between those which have been described as 'positive' and 'negative'. This distinction is important because positive disorders of behaviour are often spontaneously exhibited by an individual and occur with a relatively high frequency. Behaviours such as aggression are likely to intimidate nursing and therapy staff and prevent treatment being administered. In contrast, negative disorders of behaviour are characterised by apathy, lethargy and lack of spontaneity. These behaviours can interfere with an individual's ability to generate effort and motivation to overcome obstacles which prevent recovery and independent living. In some respects the division between positive and negative disorders is based on an understanding of the drive mechanisms which underlie behaviour.

Patients with positive behaviour disorders usually have an intact drive state with a healthy desire to achieve some form of reward and the ability to discriminate between pleasant and unpleasant consequences of their behaviour (even if such control over their behaviour is lacking). The negative disorders, however, frequently include behaviours which are characterised by their lack of motivation or incentive. Patients seem disinclined to make any effort in order to obtain the nice things in life which, in a behaviour management model of rehabilitation, may be used as rewards or reinforcers for cooperative or effortful behaviour. Whereas positive disorders often follow frontal or temporal damage, negative disorders are frequently seen following brainstem or diffuse cortical injury. They are often associated with reduced arousal, and any behaviour change that takes place as a result of direct therapy often fails to consolidate or generalise. Consequently, this category of behaviour disorder carries a pessimistic prognosis for recovery.

The final category of behaviour that has clinical significance is one in which the psychiatric components of the behaviour disorder are predominant. Eames and Wood (1981) and Wood (1987) describe hysterical, disassociative or dyshedonic disorders of behaviour as possibly being the most difficult to control and change. They are also the most frustrating to deal with clinically, because one perceives that the patients have the ability to change the behaviour in question and produce a subsequent improvement in their independence. For some reason, however, such patients 'choose' to maintain the *status quo*, often using their energies to fight against the efforts of the rehabilitation team, thereby showing that they have considerable motivation, but that it is used in a negative way to prevent progress.

A STRUCTURED APPROACH TO TREATMENT

A clear understanding of the type and nature of the behaviour disorder will facilitate the development of a treatment plan, helping to incorporate some understanding of how the patient is likely to respond, and the length of time needed before behaviour change is complete. This information is important because it directly affects the way a rehabilitation team organises its activities with respect to an individual patient.

The management of a behaviour disorder may determine how rehabilitation therapists direct their treatment towards other patients in their care. This is because the amount of time required to deal with a behaviour problem may influence the time available for other therapy activities, unless the rehabilitation team and the environment in which they work are properly organised. Before going on to discuss individual techniques, therefore, it is important to look at how a brain injury rehabilitation unit, which attempts to incorporate a behaviour management perspective into its treatment system, needs to be organised.

1. Staff training

Probably the essence of a successful behavioural management system as a model of patient care is a consistent attitude and approach to treatment by all members of staff. To begin with, the term 'treatment staff' must include nurses as well as therapists and, wherever possible, an interdisciplinary approach to treatment should prevail. If any member of the treatment team strikes a discordant note, either in respect of a particular treatment policy or in resisting the idea of working closely with another member of staff, then the successful outcome of treatment may be prejudiced.

In order to maintain a high level of staff morale and achieve an understanding of the behavioural procedures used in treatment a comprehensive in-service training programme is needed. Many behavioural procedures impose control over a patient's activities, and staff members need to be fully aware of the reasons for this control: what it is designed to achieve, how it relates to more conventional therapy and how the various reinforcement contingencies are to be implemented. Without this knowledge there is a danger of a punitive attitude developing on the part of some staff which can undermine the quality of treatment and staff–patient relationships. The two main elements of this training programme are the description and recording of behaviour, and identification of reinforcers.

2. Describing and recording behaviour

Behaviour is defined as the activities of another person that can be directly observed. These observations need to be described accurately and carefully, avoiding inferences, subjective interpretation or evaluation which can bias the observation. Because behaviour is often determined by aspects of the environment, observations of behaviour should record not just the activity but also the place and circumstances in which the activity is being observed. This may allow us to change a person's behaviour by changing the environment in which the behaviour takes place. It is therefore important to have a clear idea of how the behaviour interacts with the environment in order to formulate a treatment plan.

The process of observing and recording behaviour is usually referred to as a 'behavioural baseline' (see Sheldon, 1982 for a description). Behavioural baselines record the type, frequency and duration of specific behaviours before treatment begins, allowing a comparison of that behaviour during or after treatment with the pre-treatment baseline. A response, in order to be suitable for behavioural observation, should meet three criteria:

(a) *Objectivity*. Defining the behaviour exactly is very important. To be objective, the definition should refer only to discrete events that are directly observable. They should not include any inference about emotional state.

(b) *Clarity*. The definition should be as unambiguous as possible. The definition given should give just the right information, so that anyone reading the definition will know exactly the behaviour to be recorded.

(c) *Completeness*. The definition of the behaviour should be such that an observer will be left in no doubt as to when the target behaviour has started, and when it has finished.

Wood (1987) gives an example of the use of these principles to describe aggressive behaviour in order to discriminate purposeful and premeditated aggression from organically driven behaviour.

When recording behaviour it is important to describe aspects of both desirable and undesirable behaviour. Desirable behaviour can be described as adaptive behaviour and something which rehabilitation staff would want to encourage because it leads to a greater level of independence on the part of the patient. Undesirable or maladaptive behaviour is something which normally we would not want to encourage, either because it hinders the process of rehabilitation or because it prevents the patient being accepted back into the community and thus has implications for the patient's quality of life.

Distinct from the above behaviours is a category described as 'behaviour deficits'. This refers to a lack of social or functional skills necessary for independent living. In order to carefully identify and record the extent of these deficits it is necessary to take the patients into as many community settings as their level of recovery will allow. The presence of behavioural deficits can sometimes result in confusion because a paradoxical situation seems to arise when, as a patient is observed to improve, so the number of behavioural deficits recorded can increase. The reason for this is that during the early stages of recovery the number of activities on which an individual patient can be assessed is quite limited. Initially, assessment of behaviour is limited to what the patient can do in the unit, and this may not be compatible with the demand imposed on those same abilities when the patient is out in the community. For example, a patient may be able to understand and deal with the exchange of money in the quiet of a therapy room, but finds it quite difficult when the same exchange must take place at a check-out in the local supermarket. It is only with increasing recovery and mobility that the patient can be exposed to these different community situations and the range and extent of the behavioural deficits properly determined.

Detailed observations of behaviour allow certain 'target behaviours' to be identified. These are specific behaviours which the treatment team need to focus upon in order to improve social and functional skills that promote activities of daily living. The importance of selecting target behaviours is that many types of behaviour are made up of complex responses in which not one unit, but several units, of behaviour are linked together in some way. When behaviour change is attempted the number of behaviours that make up a complex response can be confusing, and can cause members of the treatment team to be unsure how to react or implement reinforcement contingencies. Singling out one individual response as a target behaviour simplifies the process of implementing behaviour change in a systematic way.

3. Identification of reinforcers

A reinforcer is some event which follows a behavioural response and influences that response in some way. If a particular kind of reinforcement is frequently linked with a behaviour then the individual engaged in that behaviour develops an association between the behavioural response and subsequent reinforcement. In human behavioural learning there is some debate whether this association is formed through a process of operant conditioning or whether the association is mediated by some cognitive mechanism which establishes an expectation in an individual that a certain type of behaviour will lead to a certain type of reinforcement. The arguments surrounding the conditioning versus cognitive learning debate on human social learning are complex and need not be considered here. It should be stated, however, that this chapter takes the view that there is a distinct cognitive element influencing behavioural change and attitudes towards treatment (Alderman, 1986), but in certain circumstances a more mechanical form of human conditioning will achieve the same objectives and thus cognitive mediators need not always be of paramount concern when planning a behavioural programme (Goldstein and Oakley, 1985). It is therefore important for the behavioural therapist to have a firm grasp of some of the basic concepts of theories underlying learning theory and behavioural change, because the actual implementation of behavioural techniques may have a slightly mechanical quality which does not always fully explain the purpose of the procedure.

LEARNING THEORY: INTRODUCTION TO SOME BASIC CONCEPTS

1. Classical conditioning and behaviour modification

Whilst in many ways theories of operant conditioning have been more influential in the development of behavioural techniques, some applications still purport to owe their existence to the work of Pavlov (1927) — even if the only similarity between the therapies and Pavlov's original experiments is the terminology used to explain them.

The starting point in classical conditioning is an established reflex, and this consists of two distinct elements: a stimulus, and a response that is consistently evoked by that stimulus. This stimulus is termed the unconditioned stimulus (US). In classical conditioning paradigms this US is paired with a previously neutral stimulus (conditioned stimulus or CS) until the CS evokes the same response, when presented alone, as the US did originally. The behavioural response now elicited by the CS is termed the conditioned reflex. It is possible that the use of these basic *associational* processes can make many objects, situations or behaviours more or less attractive to a patient and influence their behaviour (see Bucher and Lovaas, 1967).

There is much evidence to suggest that we may be able to explain many of the cognitive processes involved in human behaviour by reference to classical conditioning models, and this might help to explain the role of language and cognitive mediation in behavioural techniques. For instance, a number of workers have been able to demonstrate that, in humans, informing the subjects of the events that are about to occur enhances the development and extinction of classically conditioned responses (Craighead *et al.*, 1976). The theory that some aspects of language gain meaning for humans in a way similar to classical conditioning (Staats, 1968) may partially explain these sorts of phenomema, and is important conceptually in as much as it allows behaviourists to attempt to explain cognitive processes without having to step outside their own frame of reference, and thus provide a more holistic approach to the explanation of behaviour patterns. It is Staats's contention that 'in our language learning experience, certain words are systematically paired with particular emotional stimuli (p. 13). This pairing of words and emotional stimuli means that eventually the presentation of the word alone is enough to elicit the emotional response. Thus the word has assumed a meaning for us.

In the use of behavioural techniques it is important for many reasons to consider (and in fact utilise) language. This can often be done within the framework of learning theory. In some cases one can deal with inappropriate speech or language in the severely head-injured by regarding that use of language as 'verbal behaviour' and approach it in a similar way to dealing with any other form of behaviour.

2. Operant conditioning and behaviour modification

Operant conditioning attempts to describe the relationships between behaviour and the environmental events occurring before and after that behaviour. However, in the therapeutic setting we are usually concerned with manipulating the environmental contingencies *following* a behavioural event. The notion is that behaviour change is achieved by changing the consequence of particular behaviours. These consequences can be described as any one of the following: reward, punishment, omission or escape. Associated with each of these is a predicted outcome, or effect on that behaviour. These will be described in turn.

(a) Reward, in behaviour therapy, is usually referred to as 'positive reinforcement' of a behaviour, and may be expected to increase the frequency or probability of that behaviour (all other aspects remaining the same). Examples of this would be the presentation of a positive reinforcer (sweets, money or tokens, for instance) contingent upon a desired behaviour. Saying 'well done' is another example of positive reinforcement.

(b) Punishment, on the other hand, usually leads to a decrease in the frequency of the behaviour. There are a number of different punishment techniques in behavioural therapy and these will be described in more detail below. There is some debate as to which techniques actually do rely for their effectiveness on punishment paradigms (see Wolpe, 1982, p. 258), but broadly speaking most aversive techniques and some time-out procedures could be included within this category (Murphy, 1980).

(c) Omission refers to the omission of a reinforcer following a behaviour. This is generally referred to as 'negative punishment', and the expected outcome is that there will be a decrease in the frequency of that particular behaviour. Contingent removal of a pleasant stimulus or situation could be included here.

(d) Escape refers to the elicitation of a behaviour that leads to the escape from an aversive situation or event. In behavioural treatment programmes this is described as 'negative reinforcement'. Applications of this technique are not common in behaviour management. However it is this principle which explains the reason for requiring at least a short period of appropriate behaviour from a subject before removing them from, for instance, a time-out situation — to remove them during a period of inappropriate behaviour would lead to reinforcement of that inappropriate behaviour.

We have now briefly described some of the theory behind behavioural change, but before going on to look at the specific
techniques themselves in more detail, we should first look at some of the basic principles of 'extinction' — that is to say, the way in which behaviour changes in the absence of reinforcement.

EXTINCTION

The term 'extinction' refers to the process that goes on when a behaviour is no longer being reinforced. In most circumstances this means a decrease in the probability of the once-reinforced behaviour. This happens because the associations between a behaviour and its consequences, as learnt during acquisition, are being weakened. So if we are to change a person's behaviour beyond the period of the behavioural programme then it is important for us to understand the process that goes on in the absence of reinforcement.

There are four common theories of the process of extinction, and these may be described as follows:

(a) *Generalisation decrement theory.* This theory suggests that if reinforcement is omitted during extinction, responding will decline because it was not established under the conditions prevailing during extinction (Capaldi, 1967). From this we can infer that the greater the difference between what was happening during the period of acquisition of behaviour and the situation during extinction, the greater the probability of extinction. In terms of behavioural treatment, therefore, it makes good sense to conduct therapy in as many situations as possible, and if feasible, in the same circumstances as the person will experience after therapy has finished. This is most likely to enhance generalisation and decrease the rate of behavioural 'forgetting'.

(b) *Interference theory.* The response reinforced during acquisition of behaviour weakens during extinction due to competition from other behaviours or environmental events. This might suggest that both in and out of therapy it would be important to reduce this 'competition' — perhaps by increasing the salience of the ongoing reinforcers.

(c) *Inhibition theory.* This proposes that the fact of non-reinforcement in extinction is sufficient enough for subjects to learn that the previously contingent reinforcer is no longer available — in other words that the desired behaviour is no longer being reinforced. Such learning results in the suppression of the originally reinforced behaviour. It may be seen, then, that it is important in therapy to provide a positive skills-building approach, where the end-result of therapy is a situation which is inherently reinforcing and self-maintaining. The end-result of a behavioural social skills programme, for instance, would hopefully be that the subject can now interact more successfully with others. It would be hoped that this end-result should be sufficient reinforcement to maintain the behavioural learning made during therapy.

(d) *Reactive inhibition* (Hull, 1943). In the absence of reinforcement the behaviour decreases because the effort required is 'no longer worth it'. This is because there is a 'latent effort' involved in any task of behaviour. The implication for therapy is that it is not worth trying to teach a patient a new set of behaviours if, by using the old set, he/she can obtain just as large a reward for less effort. The therapy should establish a set of behaviours which enable the subject to gain more reinforcement than he/she could using the previous behavioural pattern.

The various theories of extinction are complex and largely derived from animal literature, so it is important to realise that the accounts given here are not 'pure' in as much as they are extrapolations from behavioural therapy. It must be realised that in the transition from pure laboratory theory to the human clinical situation it is impossible not to let some interpretation cloud the academic theory. But the interpretation is worth the effort, since a basic understanding of the theoretical background of behavioural therapy can greatly enhance our chances for success in the clinical situation.

Given a basic theoretical background, a more detailed description of some behavioural techniques themselves can be given.

CHANGING BEHAVIOUR: PRINCIPLES AND APPLICATIONS OF BEHAVIOURAL TECHNIQUES

Most behavioural techniques can be described as falling within one of four main theoretical categories, and these are presented in Figure 3.1. It is useful to use this as a quick reminder of the theory during consideration of the actual methods themselves. (For a practical description of the use of time-out, TOOTS and other techniques such as shaping, modelling and discriminant learning, the reader is referred to Chapter 10 of this volume.)

Figure 3.1: Basic paradigms in behavioural intervention

Technique:	Positive reinforcement	Negative reinforcement
Aims to:	Increase frequency of behaviour	Increase frequency of behaviour
Form:	Present something desirable	End something undesirable
Technique:	Positive punishment	Negative punishment
Aims to:	Decrease frequency of behaviour	Decrease frequency of behaviour
Form:	Present something undesirable	Remove something desirable

Positive reinforcement

The type of reinforcement most frequently used in clinical settings is positive reinforcement. A positive reinforcer is something which is usually considered pleasant and acts as a reward for behaviour, increasing the likelihood of that behaviour being repeated. Positive reinforcers can take the form of tangible or consumable substances, e.g. money, chocolate, soft drinks, etc., but these easily administered forms of positive reinforcement should not be used without social reinforcement, administered through different forms of attention; giving praise, encouragement or simply showing the patient that you are aware of the behaviour which is taking place.

There are two main categories of positive reinforcers: primary and secondary. Primary reinforcers are stimuli which are inherently rewarding in themselves — they do not require that the subject learn their value. In most cases desired consumable substances such as those mentioned above could be regarded as primary reinforcers. Secondary reinforcers, on the other hand, are those which have no inherent reinforcing qualities in themselves, but are reinforcing because the subject has learned what they represent. In this category one might consider money or tokens, or positive social reinforcement. In instances where stimuli are associated with many different rewards (such as money or tokens), they can be regarded as 'generalised conditioned reinforcers'.

Thomas (1968) provides a number of guidelines which he considers govern the effectiveness of positive reinforcement:

(a) The response to be reinforced must first be given, otherwise reinforcement is not possible.

(b) Reinforcement should be contingent on the response or, if not, as soon after the response as possible (when dealing with the brain-injured, contingent reinforcement may need to continue for longer than is normally expected in other clinical populations).

(c) Reinforcement of every desired response given is the most effective way of establishing a desired response pattern.

(d) Intermittent reinforcement of desired behaviour during their establishment, while less effective in achieving immediate high rates of responding, is generally more effective in producing behaviours that endure after re-inforcement is terminated. This seems to work because the periods of non-reinforcement work as a kind of 'inoculation' against extinction. This is termed the 'partial reinforcement effect' and one theory suggests that it works because it establishes associations that are appropriate for maintaining performance during the conditions encountered during extinction i.e. non-reward (Mackin-tosh, 1974). The importance of reducing frequency of reinforcement as a programme progresses can thus be seen.

(e) The stimuli suitable to reinforce one individual's behaviour may not be the most appropriate for another. We do not all find the same things rewarding, and it is important to determine the particular thing or situation which each particular subject likes before instituting a positive reinforcement programme.

Negative punishment

The withholding of positive reinforcement is referred to as negative punishment. If a person is used to a particular type of behaviour being followed by some reward, the omission of that reward may lessen the reason for displaying the behaviour. At the very least it may influence the amount of effort a person is likely to generate to produce a particular behaviour. Therefore a systematic withholding of reward for behaviour that should be discouraged is likely to gradually lead to a reduction of the strength and frequency of a behaviour and lead to its eventual elimination.

The differential use of reward or non-reward is very import-ant in controlling many aspects of behaviour. If attention is regularly given to inappropriate behaviour then there is a tendency for the frequency of that behaviour to increase, and inappropriate behaviour will occur more frequently than appropriate behaviour. The process of switching our attention (by giving some other form of systematic reward) from unwanted behaviour to desirable behaviour can sometimes increase the frequency of unwanted behaviour before it finally burns itself out through lack of positive reinforcement. Treat-ment staff should be aware of this fact if they are to have the confidence to continue a treatment programme long enough to produce any change in the person's style of behaviour.

Extinction

The 'extinction method' is often called time-out-on-the-spot or TOOTS (Wood, 1987), which probably gives a more accurate indication of its nature. Simply, it is the withholding of social attention contingent upon the undesirable behaviour. In this way it is similar to other time-out procedures, but the difference is that it is carried out *in situ*.

Many inappropriate behaviours are maintained by the attention they attract. Often the patient lacks other, more appropriate ways of attracting attention, and for this reason it is always important to use TOOTS in conjunction with contingent positive reinforcement for appropriate behaviours.

Many different types of inappropriate behaviour have been reduced using this method, including enuresis (Azrin and Foxx, 1974), stuttering (Azrin and Nunn, 1974) and abusive behaviour (Wood, 1987), but extinction methods may not always be the correct treatment choice. Murphy (1980) lists five reasons to consider before using this approach:

(a) It may be impossible to prevent the contingent presentation of the reinforcer (i.e. social attention). It is impossible to ignore physical aggression, for instance.

(b) It may be undesirable to withhold the contingent reinforcer for practical reasons. If the undesirable behaviour is leading to imminent disaster (for instance, the behaviour is severe self-mutilation) some intervention will of course be needed.

(c) The expected increase in the rate of the undesirable behaviour at the beginning of treatment may make an extinction programme inappropriate or dangerous. This phenomenon was first observed in the laboratory by Skinner (1938) and is termed the 'extinction burst' phenomenon. Where an initial increase in the undesirable behaviour might lead to added physical harm, an extinction programme might not be the most appropriate choice of treatment.

(d) Extinction may be considered inappropriate where a quick result is required, particularly if there is evidence

that the behaviour has been only intermittently reinforced (see above). Extinction methods do not always
have a quick effect, and Murphy recommends that it may
be possible to speed up the extinction process by altering
the reinforcement schedule to a continuous one before
beginning extinction.

(e) In some situations, although it may seem to be appropriate at first sight to use extinction to reduce undesirable
behaviours, practical problems may arise which would
make the use of this technique unwise. One of the
problems that Murphy foresees is where visitors to the
unit (or untrained people) might inadvertently reinforce
the behaviour with attention, even though the unit staff
are ignoring it.

In the case of using extinction with the brain-injured, Wood
(1987) gives an example of how the process might fail if the
patient's attentional abilities are not considered. Following
frontal injury, for example, we need to ensure that the patient is
actually aware of the behaviour and, consequently, aware that
he/she is not being 'rewarded' for it.

Although there is a need to consider these constraints before
employing an extinction (TOOTS) procedure, our clinical
experience is sufficient to make us confident in endorsing the
use of extinction for many behaviours which are considered to
be attention-seeking. The reservations described by Murphy
need to be placed in context and therapists must understand
that it is the *amount* of attention given and/or the quality of that
attention that is important. Obviously, a patient who punches a
hand through a glass window, lacerating his/her wrist in the
process, cannot be ignored. It is not necessary however, to
display obvious alarm at this behaviour. Staff can intervene
quickly and efficiently, providing adequately for the *medical*
needs of the patient, without any emotional display or excit-
ability. These are the reactions that maintain such attention-
seeking responses, so if staff deal with the problem in an
expeditious way, but adopt a rather indifferent or blasé manner
to the circumstances of the incident, then the emotional basis of
the behaviour is largely undermined and the 'cost–benefit' of the
self-injurious behaviour is decreased.

Similarly, the argument that visitors and ancillary staff may
provide intermittent reinforcement can also be put in perspec-

tive by staff understanding that the process of behaviour management is vastly more effective if it is carried out in a social milieu that incorporates *all* individuals who enter that milieu. This includes visitors, cleaners, maintenance men, etc. It is the responsibility of the treatment team to keep such people fully informed of the climate of behaviour that currently prevails on such a unit and ask (and expect) 'visitors' to abide by the rules of the society they are entering.

Overcorrection

Overcorrection has been defined as a procedure which requires the subject to produce a response which is incompatible with, or corrects the effects of, an undesired response (Azrin *et al.*, 1973). Practically, this usually means the repeated request for behaviours which are aimed at correcting the consequences of the undesirable behaviour. In overcorrection the individual is taught the *response costs* of a behaviour by repeated practice. Overcorrection should not be perceived as punishment: the difference between overcorrection and punishment is that in overcorrection the patient practises behaviours which are socially relevant and appropriate, as an exercise following some misdemeanour. This practice element is not a component of other punishment procedures. The target behaviours tackled using this method have most commonly included disruptive and aggressive behaviours (Foxx and Azrin, 1972) stereotyped and self-stimulatory behaviours (Azrin *et al.*, 1975), theft (Azrin and Wesolowski, 1974), coprophagy and pica (Foxx and Martin, 1975), stripping and toileting 'accidents' (Foxx and Azrin, 1973).

Procedural forms

The practice of overcorrection involves two separate procedures: restitution and positive practice (Foxx and Martin, 1975), used either separately or together. One problematic aspect of overcorrection procedures is that the activity is not reinforcing. If staff do not reinforce patients for complying with instructions during overcorrection sessions, it is less likely that the patient will perform the appropriate behaviours. To get around this problem it may sometimes be necessary to use a procedure termed 'graduated guidance'. In addition, there is a variation on the overcorrection theme termed 'required relaxation'. These procedural forms are described below.

Restitutional overcorrection

This involves restoration of the consequences of the subject's inappropriate behaviour. So in the case of someone who consistently throws meals on the floor at mealtimes, for instance, the 'restitution' might involve some 15–30 minutes of repeated 'clearing up' of messes on the floor.

Positive practice

This involves 'practising appropriate modes of responding in situations in which the subject normally misbehaves' (Foxx and Martin, 1975). In the above example of meal-throwing the subject would have to repeatedly practise the appropriate collection of meals, sitting at a table and so forth.

Graduated guidance

This is used whenever the patient fails to follow a verbal instruction (Foxx and Azrin, 1972). Graduated guidance aims to use the minimum physical 'guidance' necessary to ensure that the subject performs what is required. The idea is that staff do not force compliance through actual physical manhandling, but rather prevent any attempt the subject might make to do anything other than that which is required. In the case of our meal-thrower, for example, such patients might simply be prevented from doing anything else that they want to do until the required action is completed. The amount of guidance given is steadily reduced as cooperation increases. At the same time, verbal instructions may be given, and physical assistance is reduced as verbal control is established. The idea is that eventually the patient's behaviour will be verbally mediated without recourse to physical intervention.

Required relaxation

This procedure, which used to be termed 'quiet training', is another form of overcorrection. Following a period of behavioural dyscontrol the subject is required to go to a quiet area (a bedroom for instance) and remain quietly there for some designated period of time. Often relaxation methods can be practised in this time. In some ways this procedure resembles certain time-out methods (see below). This procedure is often applied following aggressive or explosive type outbursts

(Webster and Azrin, 1973). The rather longer duration of required relaxation differentiates it from time-out procedures, which are generally of shorter duration.

Length of sessions

It has been recommended that overcorrection sessions last from a few minutes to as long as 45 minutes. Often the length of time taken will be dictated by the subject's level of cooperation and the nature of the disruptive behaviour. The ideal duration is the shortest necessary to achieve the desired effect. In order to facilitate this, each stage of the programme must be carefully recorded. Once the patient's target behaviour is under control, the aim is to use only a verbal reminder as a way of maintaining control.

It should be noted that there is some evidence which suggests that overcorrection may actually worsen behaviour in some subjects (Azrin and Wesolowski, 1985; Azrin *et al.*, 1975; Measel and Alfieri, 1978). In addition the theoretical explanation of its efficacy lacks substance.

Differential reinforcement

There are a number of applications of differential reinforcement in the treatment of inappropriate behaviour disorders. These will be described in turn.

Differential reinforcement of other behaviours

In some cases it is not possible to switch positive reinforcement from undesirable to desirable behaviour, simply because there is not enough desirable behaviour existing at any given time. On such occasions the process of differential reinforcement for other behaviours (DRO) can be implemented. In this procedure any positive or constructive behaviour can be positively reinforced. The behaviour targeted need not be meaningful or socially important in any way; it is simply a more constructive alternative to the range of inappropriate or unacceptable behaviours that the patient is displaying at that particular time. The rationale of this procedure is that through the use of contingent reinforcement we can begin to gain control of a patient's behaviour. The degree of success achieved by this method will depend on a number of variables:

(a) Frequency of positive reinforcement will depend upon

the subject's range of behaviours other than the target behaviour. Where the range is restricted, the frequency of positive reinforcement may not be high enough to compete effectively with the problem behaviour.

(b) In practice it may not prove easy to define the behaviours which are to be reinforced.

(c) The systematic reinforcement of other behaviours requires high observer agreement, necessitating considerable training.

However, a variety of behaviours have been reinforced using this method (Allen and Harris, 1968; Bailey and Myerson, 1973; Warren and Burns, 1970) although there is little material documenting their use with the head-injured (Wood, 1987).

Differential reinforcement of incompatible behaviours (DRI)

This method reinforces behaviours which are incompatible with those we want to extinguish (Young and Wincze, 1974). Tarpley and Schroeder (1978) have suggested that this method may prove more effective than merely reinforcing any other behaviour, and this seems intuitively likely.

Differential reinforcement of low rates of responding (DRL)

Deitz (1977) has suggested that in cases that prove to be of high frequency and particularly resistant to intervention, one can initially begin by reinforcing low rates of the behaviour. It is suggested that after having been used in the initial stages, the DRL programme be converted into a DRO schedule in order to achieve complete response suppression.

Advantages of differential reinforcement methods over some other behavioural techniques are that the nature of the reinforcement paradigm is such that it is likely to prove popular with relatives and staff, and that it is possible to train relatives how to use DRO methods.

TIME-OUT METHODS

Theoretically, time-out methods rely for their effectiveness on removal of the subject's opportunity to gain positive reinforcement contingent upon the inappropriate behaviour. However it is agreed by many that time-out relies for its effectiveness on its aversive qualities. In practice 'time-out' either means removal of subjects from an environment where they can gain positive reinforcement, via a time-out room, or a time-out-on-the-spot (TOOTS) procedure, where the positive reinforcer (social reinforcement) is removed contingent upon the target behaviour. The Mental Health Act 1983 (UK) section 118 Draft Code of Practice distinguishes between three forms of time-out:

(a) *activity time-out*, where the subject is simply barred from participation in the activities by ignoring or moving away from the subject, or by steering the patient a short distance away from the activity;

(b) *room time-out*, where the subject is taken outside the room where the activity is taking place, but is aware that the activity is continuing without him;

(c) *seclusion time-out*, placing the patient in a designated 'time-out' room.

These forms and their practical application are described in more detail in Chapter 10.

The effectiveness of many of these methods may depend on factors such as the subject finding his habitual environment reinforcing, or there being a consistent expectation of reinforcement. Obviously aspects of the environment may appear reinforcing but may not be so, underlining the need for careful evaluation in each case.

There is evidence that the length of time-out episodes may be a determining factor in its effectiveness (McFarlain *et al.*, 1975) and the effectiveness of the procedure may depend upon determining the optimal time interval for each subject (White *et al.*, 1972).

Rules of reinforcement

There are some rules concerning the administration of reinforcement. The first rule conforms to the idea that it is possible to have too much of a good thing! If a positive reinforcer is presented frequently its value can be reduced, and the person receiving the reinforcement is said to have become 'satiated'. This is easy to understand if one administers chocolates as a form of reinforcement. People with normal appetites can only consume so much chocolate before what was originally an enjoyable or appetising stimulus becomes a nauseating one. The same problem is true of all consumable reinforcers, which means that a treatment programme that relies on the selective use of reinforcers should have a wide range of reinforcers to prevent satiation occurring. This choice is also likely to maintain a level of incentive on the part of the patient for as long as possible.

A second rule of reinforcement is that reinforcement is what the patient, not the members of the treatment team, sees as rewarding. For example, many members of hospital staff are non-smokers. They may dislike and object to patients smoking in certain clinical areas. If cigarettes are a potent form of reinforcement, however, then their use should not be avoided, especially if the patient is willing to make more effort for the reward of one cigarette than he is for a box of chocolates. The habit of smoking may be an acceptable price to pay for the achievement of greater independence and improvement in the quality of life for a young adult.

A third rule involves the cost–benefit of the behaviour–reinforcement exchange. This refers to the need to maintain a realistic attitude about the amount of effort we are expecting from a patient to complete a task and the value of the reward we are prepared to give in response to that effort. Few people reading this book are so altruistic in their attitudes that they are prepared to work a 40-hour week for only half the salary that their colleagues receive for doing similar work. Most people are prepared to conform to the role 'a good day's work for a good day's pay', and a patient involved in rehabilitation should not be considered an exception to that rule. It is not uncommon, however, to see nursing or therapy staff adopt a patronising attitude to patients who are receiving treatment. If this is perceived by the patient then the attitude of the member of staff acts as a punishment rather than a reward for the effort the patient is making in therapy. The adoption of a more realistic attitude can help to stimulate greater efforts on the part of patients whose brain injury has interfered with their motivation, and who are unable to generate the same enthusiasm as some other types of patient who may be receiving rehabilitation.

The final rule about reinforcement concerns the way it is

administered. There is little point in handing out tokens or other forms of reward unless it is accompanied by some form of genuine social praise, and there are two reasons for this: firstly, brain-damaged patients have often lost the social awareness to understand the significance of praise — therefore we should be re-educating them about its meaning; and secondly, often the patients will not initially be able to grasp the significance of secondary reinforcers, and by giving them praise as we hand the tokens to them, we are teaching them that they have value.

The power of the reinforcement can be determined by the time factors involved between the behaviour occurring and the reinforcement being administered. The most powerful form of reinforcement occurs when it takes place immediately following the behaviour. This is described as contingent reinforcement. Clearly it would not be possible to provide all reinforcement in this way, so an alternative is to introduce a form of interval reinforcement whereby patients are rewarded (or not rewarded) after certain intervals of time, depending upon the appropriateness of their behaviour during that time. In most behavioural procedures, contingent reinforcement is used at the start of behavioural training in order to establish a particular behaviour at a reasonable level of frequency. To maintain behaviour, however, the process of interval reinforcement is introduced, at some later stage, to control the frequency of response and prevent satiation occurring.

One way of helping the value of the reward to match the effort of the patient is to use 'tokens' to administer reinforcement instead of the consumable rewards described earlier. A token is usually a plastic disc (although in some American hospitals real money or monopoly-type money is used). These tokens acquire a value which is determined by some 'exchange rate'. For example, an individual patient may regard a visit to the local cinema as a worthwhile reward for making a significant effort on a particular rehabilitation exercise (e.g. mobility training). The reinforcement can be arranged by giving tokens to the patient at stages during therapy, when achievements are made which contribute to the acquisition of a particular skill. It may be that the value of the actual reward will be 100 tokens. The staff and the patient should then agree how many tokens should be allotted for completion of each stage in the task, a process which not only maintains effort but also gives feedback to the patient regarding the success of the efforts.

FROM THEORY TO PRACTICE: TOWARDS A COHERENT TREATMENT ORIENTATION

Whilst early behavioural therapists were inclined to adhere closely to a purely behaviouristic explanation of their methods, more recent theorists have pointed out several issues which suggest that simple extrapolation from animal experimental data to human clinical therapies is not always satisfactory (Davey, 1981). There seem to be two main reasons for this. Firstly, humans often use language to self-regulate their behaviour, i.e. people 'talk to themselves'. This means that they respond differently to animals in experimental situations. Secondly, humans live within a social environment, and many non-specific factors in both the therapeutic and the experimental situation influence the way in which they perceive both what is expected of them, and the reinforcement contingencies themselves.

The main thrust of this chapter has been to explain the process of behavioural change using a reinforcement paradigm. It must be remembered, however, that for many brain-injured patients a system of rewards is not adequate to ensure behavioural change. This is because brain damage, especially to the frontal areas of the cortex, can significantly reduce a person's sense of pleasure or idea of value that is usually intrinsic to the reinforcement-based philosophy of behaviour management. Wood (1987) attributes this to a lack of hedonic responsiveness, related to a pattern of cerebral dysfunction which implicates areas of the frontal cortex and their connections with the limbic system.

The explanation is complex, but its consequences are fairly straightforward. It means that individuals who have a diminished sense of pleasure or reward, as a result of their injuries, will not make the necessary effort to overcome obstacles in the way of reducing handicap; neither will they respond to, or value, the type of rewards generally available in a clinical environment. Basically, they seem to perceive the amount of effort needed to achieve a specific reward as being excessive to the intrinsic value of that reward (independent of the actual value).

The presence of this type of motivational deficit means that some other strategy, in addition to reinforcement, must be available to therapists engaged in the behaviour management of brain-injured patients. The most obvious alternative is to help a patient acquire a more adaptive behavioural response through the development of a 'habit'. Habits have always been recognised as a form of learning, and represent a style of behaviour over which we have little conscious control. The concept of habit is purely mechanical, and has been used to explain behaviour that had an automatic quality. Bolles (1979) describes it as a special form of stimulus–response learning which occurs primarily in the context of well-practised motor skills.

The essential assumption about habit-learning is that if a voluntary or conscious act is repeated often enough it would become attached directly to a stimulus and would no longer require awareness. Hull (1943) combined concepts of drive, motivation and stimulus–response learning to determine the 'habit-strength' of a particular behaviour. It is not possible to describe this complex interrelationship here, but Wood (1987) has shown how the concept of 'habit-learning' can be used to establish a complex chain of response, which improves functional skills in physical therapy, activities of daily living and other behaviour skills, simply by adopting certain basic principles of learning which require therapists to take account of a patient's cognitive limitations and break down a pattern of behaviour into small units, each capable of being understood by the patient and requiring a specific response. The practice of these individual units (with or without reinforcement) can help the patient acquire a range of functional behaviours and potentially avoid the difficulties encountered when dealing with patients who seem to lack the basic needs that normally drive or motivate us to achieve specific rewards.

Whilst we may not always agree that the methods we are using with our patients can always be described according to the simplistic conditioning theories above (London, 1972), what we may agree on is that the methods themselves provide a structure in which therapy can take place. The way in which the technique is used may often be as important as the choice of the 'technique' itself, for the non-specific reasons stated above. It is important, therefore, for the therapist to realise that they are just as much an agent for behavioural change as is the format of the therapy. Social reinforcement (i.e. praise or congratulation) is a powerful agent for change, and in some cases this form of reinforcement may be more salient to the patient than more tangible forms. What the techniques above all have in common is that they provide a structure and format for the presentation of reinforcement (including social reinforcement), and it is this commitment to consistency and careful analysis which often proves as valuable as the theory behind the technique itself.

4

Functional Skills Training in Severe Brain Injury

Gordon Muir Giles and Jo Clark-Wilson

INTRODUCTION

Therapists teaching functional skills need to continually evaluate their treatment approaches and their effect on the patient. Most discussions of therapeutic interventions with the severely brain-injured fail to address the issue of spontaneous recovery (see Chapter 1). Here this issue is avoided by centring most of the discussion around post-acute patients, i.e. patients in whom rapid spontaneous improvement is no longer taking place. It is hoped that these methods will also be effective early in rehabilitation. A significant proportion of patients recover without significant deficits. This chapter is, however, primarily concerned with those patients who are likely to retain significant impairments. A related question is which skills to train and when. Unfortunately no definitive answer is possible so that the timing of intervention remains a matter for clinical judgement. During the period of spontaneous improvement skills may recover at different rates, but no large group of patients has been evaluated carefully enough to provide indicators of when to become concerned about a particular skill area. Often careful monitoring of a patient's improvement will highlight where recovery has slowed, or is not occurring at all, indicating that a training approach maybe used to advantage. Where a skill deteriorates without clear cause, training may be indicated. Where persisting memory impairment is impeding progress training programmes are also indicated.

THE ACUTE STAGE AND PVS

Assessment of function and interaction with the patient begins early in recovery. If the patient is to maintain maximum motor skills, early intervention is necessary. In the acute stages of recovery the brain-injured adult can present a range of problems, such as raised intracranial pressure, decreased cerebral perfusion and electrolyte imbalance. The management of the comatose patient is largely dependent on specialised medical and nursing intervention. Where coma persists for longer than 24 hours the therapist should advise on the management of abnormal tone, splinting and positioning in an attempt to reduce tonal abnormalities, the formation of contractures or the development of pressure areas. Accepted practice is to provide passive range of motion at least twice a day on all limbs. Caution should be exercised where there is a possibility of limb or spinal damage, or raised intracranial pressure.

In a small number of patients coma gives place to a vegetative state (Jennett and Plum, 1979). The term persistent vegetative state (PVS) is used to describe this condition when it continues for months or years. After a period in coma, the patient enters a chronic state characterised by periods of sleep and waking. Patients in PVS maintain normal blood pressure and respiration, and their eyes open spontaneously in response to stimuli, but they do not follow commands nor do they attempt to communicate (Plum and Posner, 1980; Berrol, 1986).

Since the patient in PVS is medically stable, management outside an intensive care unit is desirable. Use of a purposely adapted wheelchair for a number of hours each day can help prevent many of the complications arising from prolonged confinement to bed (Shaw, 1986). It continues to be important to prevent contractures and the exacerbation of abnormal tone and pressure sores. The occupational therapist should also continually monitor the patient for changes in responsiveness (Berrol, 1986).

EARLY TREATMENT

Typically, as the patient emerges from coma, there is a period of delirium which is characterised by memory disturbance and may include agitated and aggressive behaviour which is difficult to control. The patient's speech during this time may be incoherent, rambling and indicate disorientation. After the resolution of the delirium the memory disturbance continues; during this time patients may be confused, irritable, fatuous, demonstrate poor attention to task, tire easily, and have difficulty communicating their wishes to others. Patients should not be taxed unduly, and functional retraining should be provided in a consistent manner by all members of the team. For example, when the patient is learning to transfer, the appropriate methods should be used by all hospital staff transferring the patient, and may be taught to the patient's family. Functional tasks selected for treatment should allow patients the opportunity to achieve some independence and success even where they cannot perform the task independently. For example, the therapist could support the patient's elbow while he combs his hair, or a sweater could be put over the patient's head and the patient asked to pull it down. Functional retraining should aim to utilise the abilities of the patient in a structured way so that the patient, the family and other team members can see the patient's recovery.

Behavioural learning techniques aid the learning of functional tasks. Most patients after severe brain injury have cognitive deficits which are likely to interfere with their ability to make use of current rehabilitation approaches, which relies to a large extent on attempting to stimulate the patient into recovery of function (see Ylvisaker, 1985). Before discussing the specifics of functional training techniques with the severely brain-injured, discussion will centre on the management of cognitive deficits.

MANAGING MEMORY DYSFUNCTION

Persisting memory disorders are a frequent consequence of severe brain injury. Having a clear idea of the patient's deficits and abilities will help the therapist establish an appropriate functional skills training programme. In order to understand how memory function can break down it is necessary to define some terms.

Retrograde amnesia is loss of memory for a period preceding the brain injury. The period for which memory is absent may be hours or months, or in extreme cases, years. Where there is loss of consciousness there is always some retrograde amnesia. In contrast, anterograde amnesia describes the absence of memory for the period subsequent to the brain injury. However, when this occurs immediately after injury it is described as post-traumatic amnesia (PTA) and does not imply that the impairment in memory function will be permanent. PTA appears to be part of the brain's reaction to acute insult, but its underlying mechanisms are unknown. PTA can last hours, days or weeks, and its duration has a statistical relationship to the severity of the injury (Chapter 1). During this period the patient is unable to remember day-to-day events, and subsequently demonstrates no recollection for that period of time. Recovery from PTA is evidenced by the patient becoming more oriented, remembering events and facts about his situation, and appearing more 'normal' to family and friends (Lishman, 1978). Residual memory deficits present after this period are likely to remain constant. In some cases the individual's memory does not recover and the individual is left with a severe memory disorder.

In its severest form, the 'amnesic syndrome', the patient may be incapable of performing any complex series of actions. For example patient P.D. was unable to wash. He could not remember anything for a sufficiently long period to establish any sequence in washing, and always needed prompting to initiate the task because he thought that it had already been performed.

PRACTICAL MEMORY ASSESSMENT

Psychologists have developed standardised tests to assess various types of memory dysfunction, such as the Wechsler Memory Scale (1945), Rey Auditory Verbal Learning Test (Lezak, 1976) and the Rey Osterrieth Complex Figure Test (Rey, 1959). In order to avoid a duplication of effort the therapist should be aware of the implications of these test results and consult with the psychologist in regard to the patient's ability. However, the results of tests may not reflect the patient's functional ability. The psychologist is mainly interested in the patient's memory, but the therapist is primarily concerned with how the patient functions despite the deficits. A number of practical tests can be used as an indication of the patient's memory status.

(1) Ask the patient if he is in a bus station, an airport, at home, in a church or in a hospital.

(2) Ask the patient on first meeting, and after having been out of sight for a few minutes, whether he has seen you before.

(3) Ask the patient if he knows where he is and how he arrived there.

(4) Tell the patient your name and your occupation. Ask him to repeat the information one minute, five minutes and an hour later.

(5) Tell the patient a name and a street address. Ask him to repeat it, and then ask him to repeat the information five minutes and then an hour later.

(6) Hide a motivating object (candy or a cigarette) somewhere in the room. Make sure the patient sees it and where it is hidden. Ask the patient to locate the object after a period of distraction.

(7) Ask the patient to find his way around the environment, e.g. can you go to the physical therapy room? Give directions to go from one place to another and see if the patient arrives or requires further instruction.

It is important for the therapist to practise this kind of procedure to ensure that patients are not given subtle clues, thereby invalidating the results. Significant deficits are usually quite obvious on this type of testing. More complex forms of memory impairment may only become evident on standardised psychological testing. Recently Wilson, Cockburn and Baddeley have produced the Rivermead behavioural memory test (1985) which is a standardised version of a number of these current behavioural tests.

Most functional tasks incorporate memory, and asking the patient to perform a simple functional task such as making a cup of tea or a sandwich may help to identify memory problems. Observations that are likely to indicate memory deficits when the patient is performing functional tasks are:

(1) repetitive questioning,
(2) an inability to sequence tasks in a rational order,
(3) repeating one element of a sequence,
(4) omitting tasks,

(5) forgetting where items are,
(6) forgetting the way from one place to another.

This type of testing may also demonstrate that the individual can manage complex tasks despite gross memory deficits.

OVERCOMING MEMORY DEFICITS

A great deal of attention has been directed to trying to overcome memory impairment in brain-injured patients (Wilson and Moffatt, 1984). There are a number of possible ways of addressing memory deficits

(1) Attempting to improve the patient's memory by 'practising' remembering. This has been called the 'mental muscle' approach to memory (Kim's game is an example of this type of memory practice) (Harris, 1984). There is no evidence supporting the efficacy of this type of treatment method.
(2) Internal strategies: these involve having the subject manipulate the information to be remembered in a new way. Such techniques would include rehearsing information frequently or attempting to substitute one type of memory for another if one type is less impaired.
(3) External strategies: these involve memory aids which can be used as external adjuncts to memory. Examples include notebooks, timetables and alarms, and may increasingly include the use of microelectronics.

Internal strategies

Changing the way an individual handles to-be-remembered material affects its ease of recall. A number of techniques are available that have been used effectively with patients under the supervision of a psychologist (Wilson and Moffat, 1984). The methods taught depend on the patient's specific deficits. Examples of these methods include the use of visual imagery (Patten, 1972; Moffat, 1984).

Verbal methods include first-letter mnemonics used to give

meaning to an otherwise meaningless list of words, e.g. 'Richard of York Gained Battles in Vain' to remember the order of the colours of the rainbow. More frequently used in clinical populations are methods which increase the amount of attention and rehearsal a subject gives to written information. The PQRST method described by Glasgow *et al.* (1977), is a method to aid in the retention of written information. Subjects can Preview a passage to be remembered, Question the purpose or meaning of the passage, Read the text carefully, State the information that has been derived from the passage and then Test themselves on retention.

Crosson and Buenning (1984) describe an individualised memory-retraining programme for a young man who suffered a brain injury as the result of a motorcycle accident. The patient was trained in a variety of strategies to improve recall of passages extracted from magazines, including a mnemonic strategy and questioning by a friend. The patient showed improvement over the 15-day retraining period which could not be accounted for by spontaneous recovery. Unfortunately, and in line with reports from other workers (Cermak, 1976; Gianutsos, 1980, 1981), the use of the strategy did not become part of the patient's everyday life.

Most memory-retraining procedures have stemmed from the laboratory rather than from the clinic, and have had little effect on everyday performance. Problems with the internal prosthetic systems are frequently significant enough to invalidate their use. The type of information that can be memorised by this method is highly concrete. In many cases it seems easier to teach the individual to write a list. Furthermore, evidence available suggests that even when individuals have fully mastered the techniques they do not use them.

External strategies

External strategies involve the use of external aids or cues to help the individual with a reduced memory capacity. As with internal strategies, patients who have significant memory deficits require training to use external aids. The advantage of the external aid is that it reduces the amount of information that has to be memorised: it is easier to learn to use a diary than it is to remember all the things in it. Some form of daily organiser such as a 'Day at a glance', which is divided into lines, each line covering a 15-minute period, provides further organisation. In some cases an aid can itself act as a prompt for its own use; for example an electronic diary might have an alarm built into it which attracts the attention of the user — and acts as a prompt to perform the task. There are various categories of external aids and a number of these will be reviewed.

Diaries

A diary is the most obvious type of memory aid, and one used by many of the general population. In order to use a diary to greatest effect an individual must be able to read and write and be able to extract the key elements from an action plan in order to write down the essential components. Some patients will be able to follow the instructions written in a diary but be unable to write in it themselves. A diary written in by others may still greatly increase an individual's level of independence. Problems which impede the use of a diary include poor retention or processing of verbal information, attentional problems and poor insight leading to an inability to judge when a diary may aid performance. The diary must always be stored in one place, either in a set location or on the person. One patient with an amnesic syndrome was taught to use a diary in combination with a wrist watch alarm. Staff initially wrote the patient's ward routine in the diary and the patient was encouraged to carry it with her at all times. The day was divided into 15-minute sections. The patient's watch showed the date and time and every 15 minutes the alarm would go off. At first the patient was prompted to check her diary and was praised for doing so. Over a number of weeks the patient learned what the alarm meant and could check her diary without prompting. By the end of six months she was also able to put appointments and other items in her diary herself. Less impaired individuals may have to check their diaries less frequently.

Computers and external cueing devices

Some computers have programmes which allow them to be used

as diaries. Computers are motivating, can be set up to have indices of useful information and even verbal (speech prompt) mechanisms. Harris (1984) provides a good review of aids available until 1984. With the rapid development of computer technology, aids appropriate to the needs of the brain-injured patient may increase. For example the Psion 'organiser' includes a watch, a calendar, a diary and programmable alarms (the Psion Organiser, Psion Ltd, 1985). Glisky and co-workers (1986) have demonstrated that the memory-impaired individual can acquire the information required to operate a word processing program, but needs specific training on each program and computer used.

Timetables and posters

Even the severely memory-impaired can learn some of the regularities of their environment provided it remains constant, the information is presented frequently, and is motivating. A timetable is a simplified version of a diary. Most institutions have a set routine that can be made into a timetable. This enables patients to understand where they are and what they should be doing, thus helping to relieve the patient's anxieties.

Figure 4.1 shows a timetable for an amnesic patient. It was located on his bedroom wall. For the first week staff frequently pointed it out to him, explained it to him and talked to him about it during spare time. After that time the patient was able to use the timetable to organise his week. One way of teaching needed information to a patient with a severe memory problem is to post a sign in his room. The sign should be large and eyecatching and displayed where the patient will read it frequently. It is often helpful to have the patient sign it to establish that the patient registered agreement.

Maps

Most people take orientation in space and time for granted, but some brain-injured patients have major difficulties in this area. For example it took patient P.D. 18 months to learn the location of his room (in a 16-bedded unit) and it took patient R.N. three months to learn where the shower was, despite the

Figure 4.1: J.B.R's timetable: a timetable used by an amnesic patient

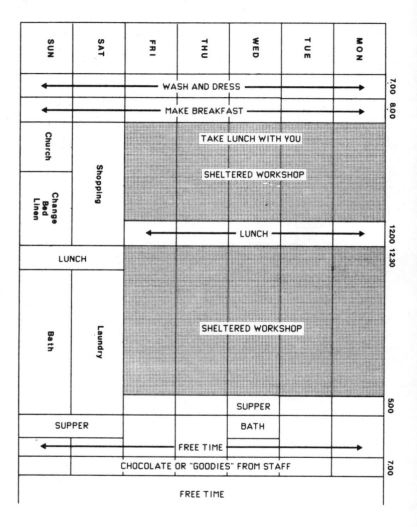

fact that it was directly opposite his room. If the patient shows poor spatial memory on initial assessment a trial should be made of how long it takes an individual to learn a specific route. If learning is not demonstrated after a number of trials alternative methods should be examined. A patient G.K. was able to compensate for an inability to recognise her environment due to central damage (her vision, though poor, was sufficient for most tasks including reading large print) by learning directions verbally ('Turn right then right again then cross two streets'). After six months attending as a day patient G.K. was unable to recognise the treatment facility but was able to use a verbal description of the facility and apply this successfully. If the problem with location is due to an apparently uniform memory deficit a map showing relevant details of the treatment facility is a simple first step in assessing the individual's ability to use a map. On a larger scale the use of a standard map and compass may be possible for some patients, but is extraordinarily difficult for patients who forget their current location from one moment to the next. For these patients a simplified map with a method of checking of each procedure as it is completed is required. A realistic aim is to teach map-reading skills and to teach future carers how to set up similar maps. For patients who are functioning at a higher level the important aspects of a complex route may be all that needs to be written down. Milton (1985) recommends the use of a card specifying the purpose, destination, bus information, landmarks to look out for and return time.

Even the most severely memory-impaired individuals can learn new behaviours if they are presented in appropriate ways. An alternative to trying to improve the individual's memory capacity is to decide what patients need to be able to do — but can't currently do — and then to train them in the activities. Goldstein and co-workers (1985) compared three types of memory training with three different amnesic patients. The patients' disorders had different aetiologies but were otherwise comparable. It was found that patients were able to learn the content of what was taught using either repetition or an elaboration method (though it was not clear that elaboration was superior to rote learning). None of the patients demonstrated generalisation of learning strategies to unfamiliar material. Patients did, however, demonstrate long-term retention of learned material. The authors interpret their results as demonstrating that the severely memory-impaired are trainable. This functional skills training will be discussed under personal and domestic activities of daily living.

ATTENTION AND INFORMATION PROCESSING

Disorders of attention are extremely complex, and a full discussion will not be attempted here (see Parasuraman, 1984, for a review). In the acute stages patients often have great difficulty in sustaining attention, and are extremely distractible. On a practical level, and particularly with the severely impaired individual, motivation is probably a significant factor. If the patient does not attend to what is being taught he is less likely to learn it. Wood (1984) has reported that patients who are undermotivated in therapy can benefit from the addition of a specific motivator such as consumables. Rather than addressing an underlying cognitive skill this is probably best thought of as 'participation in therapy', and can be assessed using behavioural measures. A test measuring behavioural aspects of attention would be a useful addition to tests available for use with the brain-injured.

For the brain-injured population a vast number of behaviours which were previously well established now require effort and attention. This is particularly unfortunate since the slowed rate of information processing after brain injury means that there is less capacity for control processing (for a fuller discussion of these issues see Chapter 7).

It may be possible to effect arousal by the use of drugs (see Chapter 2). In functional training the therapist should consider how long the patient can attend to a specific task, time of day and other variables that might affect attention. The therapist may attempt to improve the cognitive element of attention, its behavioural manifestations, or may not address attention and instead direct effort towards training functional skills. In well-designed studies which have, where applicable, made allowance for spontaneous recovery no effect of attentional retraining has been demonstrated (Wood and Fussey, unpublished data). Attempts to increase attending behaviour have been shown to be effective in various client groups, including the brain-injured (Wood, 1984; Burgess et al., 1987). Here a therapist makes a token or a tangible reinforcement, dependent on periods of time attending to a treatment session or to on-task behaviour, thereby increasing cooperation and increasing the patient's chances of learning a skill. A large number of behavioural programmes can be thought of as involving attempts to manipulate the motivational component of attention by increasing the salience of certain classes of behaviours or events for the individual concerned. For example if tangible reinforcement is made contingent on completing all the elements in a transfer programme performance levels may increase dramatically (Wood, 1984).

ORGANISATION

Many patients have difficulty in initiating actions and in their ability to plan and execute complex dependent sequences of action (actions whose performance depends on the completion of the previous action). Here the patient can benefit from training in specific required tasks.

PERCEPTUAL RETRAINING

The most frequently encountered perceptual problems after brain injury are those of visual and auditory modalities. Specialist referral is required for patients with visual and auditory problems before a realistic assessment of the patient's perceptual deficits is possible. Perceptual problems can be identified by the use of certain perceptual tests (e.g. the Rivermead perceptual assessment). Assessment of this type is only an abbreviated form of observation, and wherever possible observation on a range of functional tasks is preferable. Therapists can look for evidence of scanning problems, body schema disorders, agnosia, visuospatial deficits, left/right discrimination and colour blindness or other visual deficits.

The use of a behavioural approach allows therapists to design remediation programmes which can take into account the patient's learning difficulties. This is best accomplished in the training of functional tasks and is only described briefly here. Initially patients can be taught a behavioural response to a cue, for example, to scan left and right to the instruction 'Look'. The cue can then be used in functional settings such as in washing, finding clothes, or whilst shopping. Unilateral neglect is more common in the stroke patient than in the traumatically injured, but does nonetheless occur. Cues can be used in functional situations to address this problem. For example in training a patient with severe neglect to dress a series of prompts might include 'This is your left arm, Touch your left arm, Put your left arm into the dress' (Giles and Clark-Wilson, in preparation). Similar types of techniques can be used with patients with visuospatial disorders, dressing being a major area where performance can be severely impaired. By using auditory, visual and tactile stimuli it may be possible to 'bypass' the damaged area of the brain. For example patient M.B. had a severe receptive dysphasia, neglect, body schema disorder and right–left disorientation. During dressing training the therapist prompts M.B. with 'Give me your right leg'; if this is met with the correct response M.B. is praised and helped to put on his sock; if the wrong response is given the therapist says 'no' and taps M.B.'s right leg, then the prompt is repeated.

External aids can also be useful in assisting the patient's learning. The use of colour coding or labelling can help patients distinguish between types of clothing. This type of procedure can be used in training, gradually fading out the external or artificial aids.

FUNCTIONAL SKILLS

Activities of daily living (ADL) are probably the most important skills to be considered in rehabilitation after severe brain injury. They include those functional skills which frequently determine an individual's future living situation and hence quality of life. Some of the skills required are: (a) personal activities of daily living, e.g. feeding, toileting, washing, dressing, transferring; (b) domestic activities of daily living, e.g. preparing snacks, road safety, shopping, public transport, laundry; (c) social skills; and (d) work skills.

Deciding what functional skills to teach is influenced by the patient's learning capacity, by the individual's current level of functioning and possible future placement. Options which might raise the level of the future placement or increase the individual's level of independence within a given setting should be given a high priority. Goals need to be selected for individual patients and prioritised by the treatment team according to the patient's needs. For severely impaired patients priorities might include:

some form of purposive communication,

the elimination of serious aggressive behaviour,
incontinence,
self-feeding,
transfers,
washing and dressing,
mobility,
basic social skills.

Other goals would be more appropriate to higher functioning
patients.

EATING AND DRINKING

If coma is prolonged the patient's food intake is maintained by
total parenteral nutrition or nasogastric tube feedings. These
methods of providing food frequently continue after the patient
is out of coma, as swallowing disorders may put the patient at
risk of aspiration, or multiple injuries may have resulted in a
poorly functioning gastrointestinal tract. In the acute stages the
monitoring of swallowing is usually the responsibility of the
speech therapist and will not be discussed in detail here. The
advice of the speech therapist should be incorporated into
feeding programmes in order to aid swallowing. However, even
after the patient can swallow safely, problems may remain for a
number of reasons, i.e. the physical problems of getting food to
the mouth, problems of initiating movement and 'stuffing'
(putting too much food too rapidly into the mouth). A wide
range of useful adaptive equipment is available as a temporary
measure and may make the patient's eating considerably less
stressful in the early stages. A non-slip mat, plate guard and
wide-handled or angled cutlery may all be of use. Drinking
utensils may need to be especially light or have modified
handles. Training the patient in appropriate positioning to
maximise stability and control and decrease the effects of
abnormal tone may have significant effects on eating. Where
the physical disabilities, cognitive and behavioural difficulties
manifest themselves at meal times and persist or are particularly
troublesome, a behavioural analysis should be carried out.
    Adequate sitting balance and an erect sitting posture can be
taught in many settings either individually (Chapter 5) or in
groups (Chapter 7). As with other skills, it must be practised in

the functional setting, i.e. the kitchen or dining room. A patient, R.H. (30 months post-injury) had been taught how to use a knife and fork in conductive education sessions, but was not using these skills at meal times. R.H. was given praise if he remembered to use the knife and fork, but was otherwise prompted with 'knife and fork', which rapidly produced improved eating in the dining room.

Eating and drinking are basic skills which patients should be encouraged to perform for themselves as soon as is safely possible. Some patients can display behaviour disorders around eating which require careful management. These may be specifically related to food or evidence of wider behaviour disorders. The aim of the therapist should be to enable the patient to eat independently and safely, allowing time for adequate chewing and swallowing, and if possible, to achieve a socially acceptable standard.

CONTINENCE

If unconsciousness is prolonged patients are usually catheterised. Once the patient has the catheter removed it is important to ensure that the patient is kept dry and clean in order to avoid infection and decrease the risk of skin breakdown. Where daytime incontinence continues despite regular toileting it is appropriate to perform a medical and behavioural analysis to determine its cause. Types of incontinence include urinary retention (and overflow), reflex incontinence, stress incontinence, urge incontinence, functional incontinence and behavioural incontinence (Hartman, 1987). The first three are often the result of medical conditions arising from causes other than brain injury, such as spinal cord injury. Though all types may be seen in the brain-injured population, discussion here will centre on the general management of incontinence, functional incontinence and behavioural incontinence.

General

Bladder deconditioning may have occurred due to prolonged unconsciousness with consequent diminished bladder capacity, poor bladder control and detrusor weakness. A regular toileting programme with gradual lengthening of the periods between voids may be sufficient for bladder re-education. Starting frequency should be every two hours and twice at night (but toileting may be more frequent) with the aim to achieve a schedule of between every three and six hours. Medical and cognitive factors should be considered, which may include the effects of sedation, decreased attention to bladder cues, depression and inability to communicate needs. In planning the diet it should be remembered that alcohol, coffee and tea, and some soft drinks, have a natural diuretic effect and are bladder irritants. The therapist should establish the expectation that the patient be continent, street clothes should be worn and clothes should be changed promptly after a period of wetness to avoid sanctioning incontinence (Hartman, 1987). Adequate nutrition and bulk should be maintained so as to ensure that voiding occurs at least every three days.

Functional incontinence

Patients may be physically incapable of getting on or off the toilet, have difficulty in asking for help, or be unable to judge the time required to reach the toilet. The physical effort involved may be so great, or take so long, that patients prefer to wet or soil themselves. In these circumstances an alteration in the environment can help the patient achieve continence, e.g. ensuring the patient's bedroom is near the toilet, that the door is clearly labelled, or that the patient has a urine bottle or commode available. Patients with memory or attention deficits require prompting to assist them to learn how to manage their personal needs.

Behavioural incontinence

There are occasions when patients can be punitively incontinent as a method of showing objections to their treatment. Staff should be hesitant to adopt this formulation since the problems of coming to an accurate assessment are multiple, i.e. determining whether the problem is due to attentional deficits, memory problems, physical limitations or disinhibition. A behavioural programme aimed at increasing the benefits of continence and increasing the costs of incontinence may be useful in treating the punitively incontinent as well as the functionally incontinent patient. That behavioural intervention can be effective with even the profoundly impaired is demonstrated by a report by Cohen of work with a 27-year-old woman with encephalitis, basal ganglia damage and profound cognitive and motor involvement secondary to carbon monoxide poisoning sustained in a suicide attempt. Techniques used in treatment included *in vivo* exposure (practice), contingent reinforcement and shaping to reduce urinary and faecal incontinence, to increase toilet usage and to decrease screaming and aggression when undressed or accompanied to the toilet. Results showed a much-reduced rate of incontinence after the introduction of the programme, and reports suggest this improvement was maintained at discharge. General behaviour also showed a marked improvement (Cohen, R.E., 1986).

Night-time incontinence

In assessing night-time incontinence it is important to determine whether the patient is actually asleep. If asleep, waking the patient during the night may help him become aware of the need to urinate. Alternatively behavioural programmes similar to those used with children and described by Azrin *et al.* (1974) may be effective. Where the patient is actually not asleep simple expedients such as ensuring a urine bottle is clearly visible may be effective. Alternatively a programme of reinforcement for a certain number of 'dry' nights may be equally effective.

CASE REPORTS

Most patients respond to the types of programmes outlined above, but the following cases are particularly intriguing. Every two weeks patient P.D. (24 months post-injury) would smear faeces, tear down curtains and throw large items of furniture around his bedroom. Observation of the patient revealed that this characteristic behaviour occurred immediately before, during or after an extremely large bowel movement. Constipation continued despite the addition of large quantities of bulk to his diet. A bowel programme was initiated, in which immediately after breakfast P.D. was prompted to go the toilet, rewarded for getting on the toilet and again if a bowel movement was made. After two weeks the prompts were gradually withdrawn but reinforcement for performance was maintained. The programme was continued for 2½ months until the patient was spontaneously taking himself to the toilet. He continued to be intermittently reinforced for this behaviour. The cyclic nature of this behaviour disorder associated with constipation did not recur.

Programmes attempting to overcome incontinence arising from dyscontrol have been less successful. Patient T.M. was suffering from the long-term effects of herpes simplex encephalitis (three years post-infection) and presented a picture of incontinence arising from disinhibition and 'neglect' of bodily functions. Since the patient was very fond of music a token system was instituted. When T.M. was continent for an hour he earned a 'music token', which could be traded in for five minutes of music and other rewards. Every time T.M. was given a token he was given social praise. The importance of continence in his future life was also outlined, in an attempt to increase the salience of continence for him. When he was incontinent T.M. was asked to change and, if necessary, assisted to clear up, but no other attempt was made to increase his response costs. There was some improvement but results were disappointing. T.M. had been incontinent six or more times a day at the beginning of the programme but by the end was being incontinent once or twice per day. The change did represent a significant functional gain, but the only moderate success of this programme underlines the difficulty of working with patients whose problems are based on disinhibition. Impaired ability to make use of feedback may in part explain the uncritical attitude demonstrated by patients to their own behaviour.

Washing and dressing

In many patients washing and dressing skills return in the normal course of recovery. However, a significant proportion of the severely brain-injured do not recover sufficiently to perform basic self-care tasks independently (Weddell et al., 1980).

In attempting to remediate this deficit, each patient should be observed after being asked to wash and dress. Findings should be recorded over several days and in varying situations, and should be evaluated to assess the physical, perceptual, cognitive and behavioural deficits which hamper performance. The task requirements can then be divided into discrete steps, which can be used as prompts. Each individual programme takes into account the patient's problems and establishes ways to circumvent them. The degree to which the task is broken down depends on the individual's ability. Some patients may be able to manage with few prompts which require quite complex behavioural chains, e.g. 'Wash your face'. Other patients require the task broken down into smaller units of behaviour, 'Pick up the toothbrush', 'Put toothpaste on the toothbrush', 'Clean your teeth'. The patient can be reinforced for each item of the sequence completed. As the patient improves units of behaviour can be grouped together so that the number of prompts gradually decreases.

C.P. was admitted to the unit at the age of 37 after having suffered a severe brain injury four years before. Duration of coma was not accurately recorded but was treated in an intensive care unit for a month. When admitted C.P. had right hemiparesis involving both upper and lower extremities, poor

Figure 4.2: Graph of patient C.P's response to a training programme for washing and dressing. Open circles show prompts required to complete the task. Dark circles show the amount of physical assistance required

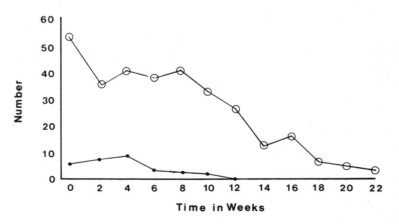

visual acuity and had poor attention, very limited speech and left–right disorientation. Memory function was very impaired. Immediate memory for digits forward and backwards was just below the normal range. Verbal memory for a short story was negligible. Patient C.P. was assessed and a programme written which consisted of 70 prompts. C.P. was told the first prompt and reinforced with chocolate and praise if she carried it out. If C.P. did not initiate the task the prompt was repeated 30 seconds later, and this procedure was continued for as long as necessary.

When the task was successfully completed the next prompt was given. Persistent comments of 'I can't' and 'Hungry' were ignored, and staff left the room if C.P. shouted, gnashed her teeth or screamed. C.P. could physically manage all of the tasks but was slow in initiating them and would always ask staff to do things for her. C.P. progressed over the next two months so that the 70-prompt system was reduced to a 34-prompt programme. This in turn was reduced to a 14-prompt programme. At this stage treatment was terminated, but when she returned to the unit six months later the skills had been maintained.

The selection of a programme depends on the individual's particular need. A programme incorporating 'assistance' can be used when the patient refuses to perform a task. The patient is prompted, and if performance does begin within a certain period the staff help the patient without any social interaction. By not performing the task the patient does not gain the reinforcement which might otherwise have been available.

A time-based programme, on the other hand, dictates the length of time under which either an individual prompt, or the entire programme, should be completed. A token programme is where a patient is given a token for each prompt completed and then can use the tokens to achieve target reinforcers, such as a magazine. All of these programmes can be designed to allow the therapist to gradually increase demands on the patient.

A programme should be gradually discontinued if the desired behaviour is to be maintained. Patient M.R. (16 years post-injury) was independent in washing and dressing when a member of staff was in the room, but if left to himself would do nothing. In order to help him retain his independence M.R. was left unsupervised, but a member of staff would drop in at random intervals and pay him a token if he was engaged in the task. M.R. needed to obtain 100 per cent token earnings for five days in order to achieve his goal, a visit to a radio station. Other targets were set and achieved, and he became independent without supervision.

Mobility and shopping

For outdoor mobility, patients need to be assessed on their ability to set appropriate goals, their knowledge of road safety, attention to traffic, ability to scan their environment and their speed of response before they can be considered safe to cross roads. Patients also need to be able to find their way to and from their destination and to behave in a reasonably appropriate manner. Some patients can walk or use a wheelchair for short distances but are unable to drive or to use public transport. Here the patient may be taught to telephone for a taxi or to find alternative forms of transport. Alternatively a wide range of outdoor mobility aids are available.

Shopping independently requires a more complex set of skills. The patient needs to have established a set of complex goals, attend to the task, find the needed items, and possess basic money skills. Patients also need to be able to handle the difficult physical tasks required in shopping, or have social skills appropriate enough to seek assistance. The planning of the patient's treatment is dependent on the expectations of the patient, the patient's family, and the therapist as well as the physical, cognitive, behavioural and social needs of the patient.

C.G.'s wife was determined to take C.G. home for weekends and out into the community, despite the fact that he was extremely verbally abusive and physically aggressive. On assessment it was noted that the inappropriate behaviour was most pronounced when the patient was in a noisy and threatening environment, e.g. near a road with traffic (C.G. referred to crossing the street as 'another opportunity to dice with death') or in a highly stimulating environment e.g. the supermarket. A programme was devised for C.G. to reduce his inappropriate behaviour. C.G. was initially taken out in his wheelchair for short distances in the hospital grounds. Then he was gradually introduced to more stimulating situations: the hospital shop and a local department store. At the same time

work was continuing on his walking, so that he was able to walk short distances by the road. When C.G. could do this without undue complaint, staff would walk with him to the hospital coffee shop. This involved crossing one of the hospital's roads, walking a hundred yards, ordering tea or coffee and finding a seat. To begin with a member of staff would walk with him, but after C.G. had demonstrated competence on a number of occasions staff became 'busy' and met him at the coffee bar.

The programme continued in this way until C.G. was able to walk half a mile to the local shops, a journey which involved crossing a number of major roads. The entire programme took four months. C.G.'s wife reported that when at home at weekends C.G. was able to go out with her to the cinema, and was able to walk by himself to the local shops.

As indicated by the results of these programmes, patients with physical, cognitive and behavioural deficits can overcome considerable handicaps if retraining is structured in such a way that they can make use of it.

To develop shopping skills training should be structured to the individual's needs. For example patient H.G. had moderate memory problems, a severe nominal dysphasia, and a left homonymous hemianopia. H.G. had not learned to compensate for his visual defect spontaneously and therefore had difficulty finding objects in his environment. H.G. also had difficulties in putting objects into categories, e.g. he knew what an orange was but he did not know that it was fruit, and he knew what a steak was but did not know that it was meat. These problems were most evident whilst shopping. H.G. could not ask where things were because of the dysphasia, he did not know where particular items were because of the category problem, and he was poor at searching his environment because of the scanning difficulties. Initially he had to be taught that he had a scanning problem, and a scanning programme was begun in the kitchen since this area also presented major difficulties. H.G. was taught a verbal prompt 'scan up, scan down, scan left, scan right' as a behavioural cue. This was extended to finding objects around the kitchen, and then was practised in a variety of other settings such as the grocery store and crossing roads. It was necessary to have H.G. repeatedly practise the skill until it ceased to be an effort. By the end of the programme H.G. was doing his own grocery shopping.

Kitchen skills

Establishing the likely level of future independence will help the therapist prioritise the patient's needs in the kitchen and establish a training programme taking the patient's deficits into account. Young adult males (a group over-represented in the brain-injured population) frequently have little or no experience in the kitchen. Patients may need to learn a number of different skills, including menu planning, organising and sequencing tasks and instruction in the use of equipment, e.g. an electric kettle or a microwave oven.

Patients with severe physical deficits can be taught to position themselves optimally to increase function and reduce the effects of spasticity. Labour-saving devices should be used with circumspection and should not be used in place of correct positioning. Often the use of aids is as difficult, if not more difficult, for the patient to learn than are new strategies for coping with his or her environment.

J.B.R. was very keen to improve his cooking skills. This was

Figure 4.3: This figure records the progress of JBR in learning to make his own breakfast. A = food and instruction sheet and additional prompts when required (primarily 'check instructions'). B = With instruction sheet, food left out. C = Without instruction sheet, food left in cupboards.

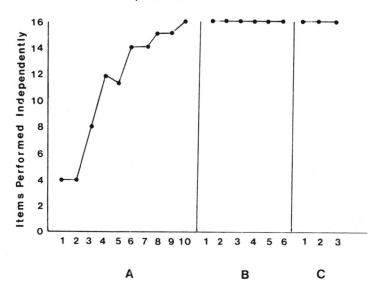

a realistic goal for his rehabilitation programme but presented particular problems for J.B.R. because not only did he have an amnesic syndrome, he also had a specific category-naming problem for foods and objects in the kitchen (Warrington, 1981). For example, J.B.R. could not distinguish food from non-food items reliably, did not know where food could be stored, what colour toast should be, what boiling meant and so on. J.B.R. could not recognise the oven or the grill or other kitchen items. J.B.R. was trained to make his own breakfast of a tin of baked beans and sausages on toast. A programme was devised, after he had been observed for a week using a set of instructions. J.B.R. was prompted with 'check instructions' on entering the kitchen. All the food items to make breakfast were set out on a tray with a copy of the instruction sheet and a pen. Any implements the patient had to find himself. The patient would tick off each step as it was completed. For the first two weeks, even with the instructions, the patient continued to make mistakes, but by the end of the third week he was independent with the instruction sheet and supervision was withdrawn. After performing the programme every morning for six weeks the instruction sheet was withdrawn and J.B.R. continued to make his breakfast independently.

It was another six weeks before the patient knew that he could make his own breakfast. This learning without awareness is frequently noted in amnesic patients. Figure 4.3 shows the course of J.B.R's learning. J.B.R. was taught to make himself other meals using similar techniques, and was also able to learn to do his own shopping and laundry with a concomitant rise in self-esteem.

All functional tasks should be taught in the most appropriate setting, which should be made as conducive as possible to learning. Although this chapter has only concentrated on a limited number of functional tasks, these procedures are capable of being applied more widely. A behavioural approach helps therapists observe and identify areas of skill and dysfunction, in the designing of intervention strategies, and provides recordings which allow realistic programme evaluation.

SOCIAL SKILLS

Despite increasing interest in interpersonal skills in the brain-injured population there are surprisingly few published reports of treatment. Nevertheless a variety of procedures have been reported, including social and tangible reinforcement, time-out (Wood, 1984) and modelling (Edelstein and Eisler, 1976). These have been used effectively in a number of populations including the mentally retarded (Bates, 1980; Bornstein *et al.*, 1980) and chronic schizophrenics (Bellack *et al.*, 1976). Studies have demonstrated the effective application of learning principles in modifying both verbal and non-verbal components of speech as well as its content.

Trower *et al.* (1978) suggest that a person can be regarded as socially inadequate 'if he is unable to affect the behaviour and feelings of others in the way that he intends and society accepts'. Many individuals with brain injury fall into the category of socially inadequate, even though they were socially skilled prior to injury. Brain injury, especially damage to the frontal lobes, may produce behaviours and emotional responses that are incompatible with acceptable social interaction (Oddy *et al.*, 1978). Lishman and others (Lishman, 1978; Lezak, 1978) have noted that adequate social behaviour is often the first thing to be impaired after brain injury. Such individuals can be self-centred and intolerant, have difficulty changing from one topic to another, and are often unable to understand abstract concepts. Not surprisingly, therefore, many brain-injured patients find difficulty in verbal and non-verbal interactional skills, such as turn-taking, meshing, listening and following changes of topic in a conversation. Bandura (1969) emphasises the importance of being able to discriminate relevant aspects of the environment in order for social learning to take place. Not only are patients unable to use environmental cues, they seem to have difficulty noting the central features of their own behaviour.

It is essential to view patients in relation to their previous personality, and their family and social setting. Assessment should include observations of how patients respond to their family, staff members, other patients and total strangers of both sexes. Conversely, it is important to assess how the patient's behaviour affects others.

The general model described for social skills training is that of Trower *et al.* (1978). Social skills are analysed, broken down into component elements and practised. Here three types of intervention are described for use with patients of different degrees of impairment. The first type of intervention is used with the severely handicapped population and concentrates on non-verbal skills. The second type of intervention concentrates on teaching basic verbal and non-verbal skills used in social routines, and then in generalising these to the realistic setting. The third type of intervention aims to help the less impaired patient learn appropriate methods of dealing with problems that are likely to occur in the community. These types of interventions will be discussed with examples below.

Level 1

The severely handicapped group includes those with major physical impairments who have little or no usable language. These patients may have problems in comprehending the type of cues that people use to understand interaction — such as facial expression — and have similar difficulties in producing non-verbal communication. Patients can often be taught the importance of these non-verbal forms of communication and how to incorporate them in their normal behaviour. Non-verbal skills include facial expression (smiling is especially important), posture, gesture, eye-contact, proximity to others and body orientation. As many patients can make sounds (voice) without being able to produce language (words) issues surrounding volume, tone, pitch and rhythm are also addressed.

An 18-year-old man, I.D., was admitted to the unit four years after his severe brain injury. I.D. possessed no recognisable language, sat slumped in a chair, and drooled constantly. When he was not given what he wanted he would scream. Many of those around him found it difficult to interact with him because of their feelings of disgust. A possible placement for I.D. had been arranged provided there were a number of changes in his behaviour. These changes included improved social skills, which was therefore regarded as a priority. Social skills training was started in a group with three other patients with similar problems. Appearance, facial expression, posture and lip closure were stressed. The importance of good social presentation was explained and practice in basic non-verbal routines begun. Patients were encouraged to sit well, with lips closed, and to voice briefly using appropriate volume and pitch, in order to attract attention. They were requested to maintain eye-contact while asking a question (by use of gesture). On all these points I.D. needed instruction, but he learned quickly and prompts were gradually phased out as he improved.

The group then worked on learning and using social routines, 'Good morning', 'Please' and 'Thank you'. The patient was taught to sit well, look and orient himself towards the person, voice and smile for 'Good morning'. A similar procedure was used for 'Please' and 'Thank you'. When these were reliably and appropriately being said in the group setting I.D. was asked to use the procedure in the ward setting. For a week I.D. was prompted in the use of the routines and praised whenever he used them. After the first week, I.D. was no longer prompted, but praise and intermittent tangible reinforcement were provided contingent on good performance. Requests which were accompanied by screaming, or were in some other way inappropriate, were not responded to. I.D. was able to maintain his improved performance, and has become socially acceptable to such a degree that staff who previously avoided him began to actively seek his company.

Table 4.1: Level 1

Non-Verbal	Verbal
1. Facial expression	1. Volume
2. Posture	2. Tone
3. Gesture	3. Pitch
4. Gaze	4. Clarity
5. Personal Space	5. Pace
6. Appearance	6. Speech disturbances
7. Orientation	

Level 2

The second type of intervention can be used with the slightly less handicapped. The organisation of the social skills session needs to take into account the patient's attentional and memory handicaps. Patients require structure and consistency to help them learn. This means that the subjects to be taught need to be repeated many times in a session and the same type of approach used each time. A dynamic and enthusiastic approach to retraining is essential, and training should take place in short 10–15-minute bursts to maintain the patients' attention and motivation. The social skills training can sometimes be incorporated into social games to make the sessions more enjoyable.

Patients often require training in how to approach people, and how to converse in social situations. They may need to be taught how to attract attention, ask simple questions, listen to people, take turns in conversation and may also need to learn to initiate and maintain conversation. These tasks can be analysed into verbal and non-verbal components and practised. For example the elements of attracting attention can be seen as:

(1) saying a person's name, saying 'Excuse me, please', or voicing (if appropriate) to attract the attention of the person they are talking to;

(2) once the person's attention is gained, the patient is taught to face the conversation partner, look at him/her (i.e. gain eye-contact), and smile.

These elements of attracting attention can be extended to include conversation management. Patients are taught how to initiate a conversation, ask questions, take turns in conversation and to maintain conversation. Finally they are taught appropriate ways to end conversations. To generalise the skills it is necessary to gain mastery in the session, then in role-play situations, e.g. in mock-up shops, and then in the real situation. Until the final stage is reached the training is not necessarily effective. This form of social skills training is very structured in the way the patients work through situations.

Table 4.2: Level 2

1. Introduction and exit skills
2. Initiating social interactions
3. Apologising
4. Situation-specific routines (e.g. shopping, telephone)
5. Accepting criticism
6. Asking for information and requests
7. Content of speech

Level 3

Patients with less severe handicaps need to learn to be flexible, reason out methods of coping with their changed lifestyle, and relearn how to socially interact with people appropriately. Patients at this level frequently have an unusually egocentric frame of reference, and need to be taught to act as if they had more interest in the needs and feelings of others. Patients at this stage in their rehabilitation programme learn to take the initiative in personal encounters, to work within and to lead a group. Subjects discussed include skills which will aid return to the community; listening and conversational skills, the giving and receiving of compliments and criticisms, assertiveness training, and skills pertinent to the needs of the group (see Table 4.2). This group can learn through trial-and-error and directional training in role-plays and functional settings, with subsequent discussion and evaluations of their performance.

R.H. was a patient who responded to any direction or criticism by moaning and justifying his actions. R.H. took instructions literally, got very anxious, and this proved to be a problem in his rehabilitation. In social skills the fact that R.H. moaned was discussed; he apologised for moaning and said he would work on it as a problem. R.H. was asked if he felt the staff could help him remember this. In response he asked if everyone would say 'Moaning' to him whenever necessary. This programme was followed, and after two weeks staff were finding him more pleasant company and more responsive in treatment.

Table 4.3: Level 3

Conversational Management

1. Content of speech
2. Listening (observing)
3. Accepting criticism
4. Assertion skills
5. Awareness and responsiveness to needs of others
6. Turn-taking
7. Giving instructions
8. Initiating social interactions
9. Apologising
10. Self-disclosure (expression of emotion)

A patient may display a social skills deficit of apparently organic origin, but this does not mean that it cannot be affected by social skills training. One patient seen by the authors had paroxysmal outbursts of swearing. The patient would apologise and seem genuinely remorseful, but be unable to stop the behaviour. A range of problems can manifest themselves as social skills deficits, e.g. lack of insight, denial of problems, sexual disinhibition or an inability to understand social norms. Patients are often unable to set themselves goals, or may set themselves unrealistic and poorly developed goals. These problems have to be carefully monitored and their learning ability recorded to evaluate the effectiveness of the training.

WORK SKILLS

It is essential the therapist gain a thorough understanding of the job requirements via a visit to the worksite, so that an analysis of the work requirements can be performed. Jellinek and Harvey (1982) found that active counselling and help in pursuing job resources significantly improved the rate of employment in a series of brain-injured patients seen in a medical facility. Patients in a higher socioeconomic class may find returning to work easier, since their jobs are likely to offer more flexibility and potential for passing responsibility to subordinates (Binder, 1986). Some patients will have predominantly physical handicaps which stand in the way of employment, and here the therapist can consult with both the patient and the employer in how the work environment might be adapted to suit the patient's needs. Many patients who return to work find that they become excessively tired, are easily distracted and have problems remembering information. Initially returning to work for half-days two or three days a week may serve not only to prevent the patient from being overtaxed and disheartened, but also to prevent the employer from making a premature judgement about the employee. It is valuable if the therapist prepares the patient for the fact that sustaining a day at work may be considerably more difficult than before the accident. Slightly altering the requirements of the job, or the addition of certain prosthetic aids, can help patients return to work despite severe memory impairments (Gianutsos and Grynbaum, 1983). Arranging the environment to reduce memory demands, the use of a notebook and setting up routines may be helpful.

A number of single case reports suggest that personality

changes after severe injury may leave the patient sufficiently able to live independently but unable to perform at their previous job (Damasio, 1985). Although many patients fervently wish to return to work, particularly their previous employment, this is often an unrealistic goal. A wide range of factors may prevent return to work; often these occur in combination. The following areas need to be assessed:

(1) physical ability and disability;
(2) cognitive dysfunction — memory, attentional, perceptual;
(3) mood disorder, disorders of drive, personality change and paranoia and obsessionality;
(4) behaviour disorders — aggressiveness, disinhibition.

Where return to previous employment is not possible vocational retraining should be considered.

Taking histories of premorbid functioning will indicate at what level the individual functioned prior to injury. Some individuals have very poor premorbid work habits, and it is unlikely that this will have improved as a result of the injury. A school, work and social history is required. Where the severity of the patient's impairment prevents a return to open employment industrial rehabilitation may be valuable.

The aims of the industrial therapy can be directed either to learning work skills or to making the patient more manageable in the community. In the short term these may not be mutually exclusive. Patients may need to learn work skills — to be able to get themselves to work — work at a steady pace — take direction and so on. Development of these skills may mean that an individual may be able to progress to a sheltered workshop and eventually to open employment. To describe industrial therapy as a management strategy is not to demean its importance. If an individual can develop and maintain sufficient control to be able to attend a day centre, industrial therapy or sheltered employment for a large part of the day, he may be able to obtain a placement which provides a much higher quality of life (e.g. home as opposed to a psychiatric hospital). Work may also integrate and reinforce the functional skills previously taught. For example patient C.G. (previously described) vastly improved his walking ability under the demands of return to work. Patient J.B.R., who had previously been taught to wash, dress, make his breakfast and find his way around, had to considerably improve his performance in order to get to work on time. Earning some amount of money and having a proper job must contribute to the patient's feeling of self-esteem.

Patients frequently find it difficult to tolerate changes in routine, interaction with co-workers, taking direction and accepting that their level of performance and competency is now considerably reduced. It is important that the work the patient gains should be suitable. For example patients working with machinery should be able to manage the job safely. If there is any doubt (especially in cases of patients with seizure disorders) the approval of the physician in charge is required.

Unfortunately some patients who have severe physical and psychological sequelae may be physically incapable of even the simplest assembly work, and cognitively too disabled for more complex tasks.

Non-work-related activities

Where full- or part-time employment (open or sheltered) is not possible the therapist should consider what other activities may be practical and appropriate for the individual, and help the carers structure the patient's day. Contact with agencies in the patient's home area should indicate the existence of, and the patient's eligibility for, day programmes. Severely impaired patients benefit from a life of structure and regularity. Where this cannot be provided by the exigencies of a working day it can be imposed by way of a routine. The patient should participate as much as possible in self-care activities. Patients may also participate to the extent of their ability, and in accordance with the need for safety, in meal preparation, shopping, house-cleaning and other activities of daily living. Patients can feel that they are making as much of a contribution as they are able, and this helps the care-giver maintain a positive attitude towards the patient. However, since fun is important the therapist should have identified and helped to develop a range of leisure interests. These might include special subjects, games, art or craft activities, sports (independently or with clubs such as riding for the disabled) and educational or leisure activities such as movie- going.

5

Rehabilitation of Physical Deficits in the Post-acute Brain-injured: Four Case Studies

Jennifer Hooper-Roe

Physiotherapy texts often divide disabilities into categories such as ataxia, spasticity and flaccidity, which are considered as individual items. This does not take into account how these separate physical disabilities combine and affect the whole person and real world functioning. The severely brain-injured person can have a multitude of physical problems, but it is the overall functional loss which is the central factor to be considered.

In addition to the brain-injured person's physical disabilities, other factors such as behaviour disorders, memory deficits, poor drive and motivation may all interfere with function. These problems have invariably been compounded by months or years of inappropriate placement and rehabilitation.

This situation presents a seemingly impossible task in starting with the rehabilitation process. Regular and thorough assessment is vital, both to evaluate the person's disabilities as a whole, and to highlight particular problem areas which can be worked on as priorities. Continual re-evaluation of treatment will demonstrate if the treatment is appropriate and achieving its aims.

In dealing with mixed physical and behavioural problems, however important each therapist regards her particular priorities, these must take second place to working with cognitive and behaviour disorders. It is these disorders that have often made previous attempts at physical rehabilitation unsuccessful so that the patient has never reached full potential.

When determining treatment priorities it is essential to consider that the patient may have impaired powers of concentration and attention. The patient may only be able to process one item of information at a time, and may only be able to cope with one area of rehabilitation at a time. For example, if a person's physical priorities are to sit well so that he can feed effectively, the initial priority may be to concentrate on sitting well. Likewise, the therapist should take into account the way instructions are given. Are they presented in such a way that they are easily understood? This can often be achieved by giving a series of one-word prompts rather than full sentences. For the person with severe memory deficits it may be necessary to break an overall treatment programme into very small items and to repeat a few simple tasks over and over again until they become automatic before being able to progress any further with the treatment programme. The physiotherapy assessment may usefully be a combination of a scoreable assessment, and a qualitative assessment looking at posture, balance and gait, fine motor control and any other significant factors. These might include swallowing and feeding difficulties, physical deformities or disorganisation of movement. The scoreable assessment deals with locomotor ability, an assessment of abnormalities of muscle tone, joint position, sense and superficial and deep sensation.

With behaviourally disturbed patients it is often not possible to gain enough help and participation from them to fully complete the assessment, and it may be many weeks of careful observation which reveal the true extent of the physical disabilities and functional deficits.

Only when as much information as possible has been collated can one then decide on which problem is a priority, and set out the aims and goals of the treatment programme. Where behaviour disorder is a factor a behaviour management system can help with this aspect of treatment (for example, see Wood, 1984; Eames and Wood, 1985b). Treatment programmes must be tailored to an individual's needs in order for them to be of the most advantage, and to make the maximum and most effective use of the treatment time available. Whilst group work has an important part to play in an overall treatment programme, particularly when a number of people need to be taught the same skill, such as sitting posture, it cannot take into account every individual's specific needs and requirements. Nor is it possible within the confines of a group situation to reinforce a desired behaviour from an individual every single time that behaviour occurs, essential where an individual has problems in new learning. Also, certain problems do not easily lend themselves to group work, such as walking or standing, when often a 'hands-on' approach is necessary.

In an individual treatment programme the treatment is tailored to the person's own unique needs, and reinforcement can always be contingent on a described behaviour every time that it occurs. There is also no opportunity for other patients to give positive reinforcement to any inappropriate behaviour. The benefits of individual treatment programmes will be illustrated in the cases studied later in this chapter.

The treatment programme needs to take into account functional activities used by the person on a day-to-day basis. For example, a person who has been working on gait re-education and fine motor control in physiotherapy sessions might be involved in outings to local shops where the main aspects of his individual therapy sessions can be focused on. The patient will need to be able to walk down a street, or around inside a shop, will also need the fine hand control needed to get money out of his pocket and then select the right amount of money. The patient can also be given the opportunity to practise the skills he is learning in treatment sessions, but more importantly he is taking part in a normal, everyday activity. It will also be far more rewarding than practising walking in the physiotherapy room and sitting at a table picking up different-sized coins. Other examples of this kind of use of functional activity could be given as gardening — where balance, walking, bending, kneeling and hand control can all be practised, or horse riding — where, again, balance and hand control are vital skills. Hopefully, too, these activities provide pleasure and satisfaction for the patient who may be unaware that he is actually practising what he has been working on in more formal physiotherapy sessions.

Whatever skills a person acquires in an individual treatment programme he should be given every opportunity to practise those skills functionally, and to be able to generalise them into different situations.

The following studies exemplify the treatment of patients with physical and behavioural problems. The actual physical treatment programmes illustrated are part of an overall treatment programme, and should therefore not be considered in isolation. They show how particular functional problems can be dealt with despite their association with behaviour disorders.

CASE REPORT ONE

S.C., a 27-year-old female, was involved in a road traffic accident in which she sustained a severe head injury predominantly affecting the brainstem. In addition to left temporo-parietal damage she also sustained a fractured left femur and a partial dislocation of the left side of her pelvis, and fractured vertebrae. She was left with a severe left-sided hemiplegia, and loss of speech. Myositis ossificans developed in the left hip which became fixed.

One year after injury S.C. was described as being totally dependent on 24-hour nursing care. She was still being fed six-hourly by a nasogastric tube, and was unable to stand or walk but could propel herself in a wheelchair. She was very poorly motivated and she sat with her head hanging forwards, tongue protruding and dribbled constantly. Any attempt at having her engage in activity was met with furious outbursts of screaming.

It was decided that the first priority would be to tackle the problems she had with swallowing and feeding and therefore a feeding programme was designed, using contingent reinforcement. This programme was performed by a speech therapist and a physiotherapist, concentrating on lip closure and movements and positioning of the tongue, and also correct posture, and efforts to initiate the swallowing reflex.

Initially S.C. was supported in a semi-reclining position with her head supported by pillows in a mid-line position, and work was begun on desensitising the lip and mouth area. At this stage the mouth was hypersensitive. Desensitisation was achieved by introducing various tastes, textures and touch to the affected area using glycerine swabs, wooden spatulas, minute quantities of sweet sauce, and ice. This procedure was necessary first to enable attempts to feed her and complete an oral toilet. In addition to this desensitising programme S.C. was given combined speech therapy and physiotherapy sessions working on posture, and movement of the lips and tongue.

In the feeding programme every attempt at swallowing was reinforced with attention and social praise, whether the swallow was purposeful or just a reflex. Swallowing rapidly improved, and small quantities of soft food were introduced. At this stage advice from the dietician was vital on which foods should be offered, taking into account the ease with which they could be swallowed, and to offer as much taste and variety as possible so that feeding could be a pleasurable event.

As purposeful swallowing improved therapists only gave reinforcement to this and ignored any reflex swallowing. As the programme continued, reinforcement became dependent on S.C. making an attempt at chewing the food in her mouth, moving it back and swallowing it. Whilst this programme continued the nasogastric tube feeding was reduced, equivalent to the amount of mashed food that S.C. was being offered at each feeding session. Again, the help of the dietician was invaluable in calculating the amount and variety of food that was offered.

Very careful documentation was used throughout the feeding programme and records obtained to show results. This was based on the following scoring system:

Score = 1   chewing and purposeful swallowing,
Score = 2   purposeful swallow only,

Figure 5.1: Improved swallowing in a patient who had been maintained on a nasogastric tube for two years and who refused to attempt to swallow. Progress rated on a 1–6 scale where 6 = no effort and 1 = purposeful swallow (taken from Wood, 1986a)

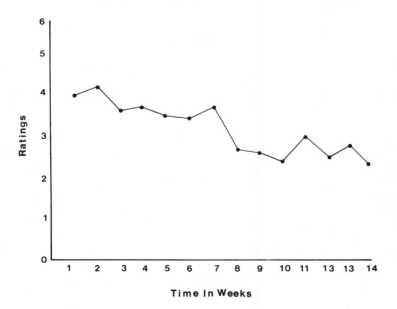

Score = 3   reflex swallow with minimal food loss,
Score = 4   reflex swallow with substantial food loss,
Score = 5   no swallow — food dribbled out of sides of mouth,
Score = 6   purposefully spitting food out.

Entries in the clinical notes during this period included the following:

June   During tea time S.C. picked up a jam sandwich, bit a piece of it, moved it around her mouth then spat it out. She repeated this until the sandwich was finished.

July   Feeding programme going well. She now assists by putting the fork into her mouth. She is only having one nasogastric feed a day and the rest of the time is being fed a softened diet in the dining room.

August   S.C. is now feeding herself with a minimum of prompts. She holds her head up and swallows effectively.

In just over three months S.C. was feeding herself satisfactorily after being fed by nasogastric tube for 2½ years.

S.C. gained a great deal of reinforcement from all the attention she received when being fed by nasogastric tube. Therefore when the feeding programme was started, being fed by nasogastric tube was done in silence, giving her as little attention as possible to decrease the reinforcement attendant upon it.

CASE REPORT TWO

C.G. had been involved in a head-on collision while driving a car in May 1983 and suffered a severe head injury. He was unconscious for seven weeks, and had a residual left-sided hemiplegia.

Initially he made good progress despite his excitable behaviour, and as the weeks progressed the residual hemiparesis became quite mild. However, C.G. became increasingly more aggressive and began to assault staff and then fellow-patients. This behaviour escalated to such a degree that it could only be controlled by large doses of sedative drugs, which left him unable to cooperate with any kind of rehabilitation procedures.

On admission to a rehabilitation unit 10 months after injury, C.G. was unable to walk but could propel himself in a wheelchair. He was extremely demanding, very noisy and disruptive. He kept up a more or less constant barrage of repetitive questions and comments, which seemed to be his way of keeping others at a distance and making it almost impossible to do anything with him. He responded very well to a time-out programme for his aggression, but any meaningful therapy was severely disrupted by his demanding behaviour and the constant flow of verbal abuse and repetitive conversation.

Physically, C.G.'s main problems were those associated with his hemiparesis. He had great difficulty taking any weight through his left side, there was increased muscle tone in both the left arm and leg, and there was no voluntary movement in his left ankle and toes. Coordination was impaired on the left side. He also had problems with functional use of his left hand. It was decided that the main priority physically was to try and get him walking, and a walking programme was started.

C.G. could stand unaided, but his balance was very precarious and his agitated behaviour was enough to cause him to fall easily. Initially physiotherapy was aimed at increasing his ability to balance in all positions, to take weight through his left side and to increase his awareness and use of his left side. He had plaster of Paris applied to his left lower leg to allow him to take weight through the foot in a corrected position. This was not very successful and so was followed some weeks later, more successfully, by a below-knee caliper. Despite his constantly noisy, uncooperative behaviour, particularly in group sessions, he made significant progress in all his major physical problem areas.

For his walking programme C.G. was given a rollator frame to assist him. In all attempts to cut through the constant tumult of chatter and abuse, verbal regulation of his actions was used very loudly and firmly by the physiotherapist. The instructions given were: 'push, step, stretch', to which he pushed the frame forwards, took one step and then straightened up. After each correct sequence he was praised profusely and given lots of attention. He responded well to this, and after a few days C.G. was encouraged to use the verbal regulation himself, which he did, but it interjected a great deal of repetitive chatter and verbal abuse. After a few days of doing the walking programme twice daily the prompt words were changed to 'one, two, three', in an effort to promote more rhythm in his gait. Within two weeks of starting this programme C.G. was walking a distance of 100 yards using the rollator frame and prompting himself with 'one, two, three'. He was also inhibiting all other language whilst he was walking.

As a progression in the programme C.G. was encouraged to think of the prompts, but not to say them aloud. Within another week he was walking the same distance in total silence. Three weeks after this C.G. was walking independently around the unit with the rollator, and only using his wheelchair outside.

Then, in physiotherapy sessions, C.G. was given a short wooden baton to hold horizontally in his hands with his arms stretched forwards fixing his shoulder girdle. The rollator was discarded for the walking programme, but in the meantime C.G. started walking outside the unit with the rollator. In the walking programme verbal regulation was used again, this time the prompt being 'step, stretch' as he took one step and straightened up. The same sequence as before was used, 'step, stretch' became 'one, two', and this in turn was internalised. Because C.G. sometimes used the baton as a weapon it was taken away, and he repeated this part of the programme using clasped hands.

Coinciding with C.G's ability to walk in this way, an event occurred which hastened the decision to take the rollator away from him for walking in the unit. During one particular walking session C.G. just walked off with his hands clasped, so it was felt he was quite able to walk without the rollator, and it was taken away for good, except for walking outside.

Progress continued and the programme was generalised into other situations. Trips to the local town were made first using the rollator, and then without. C.G. was encouraged to join in a gardening project where he was expected to manage all the necessary walking without any assistance. He was very motivated by his own success and his increased mobility spurred him on to try activities that he had previously refused to do. However, this generalisation procedure was not without its problems. With the introduction of each new situation C.G. became very excitable and noisy and it was often necessary to use prompting again, and go through the sequences used at the start of the walking programme to help him overcome his agitation.

Physiotherapy continued in many other settings — for

example, in the kitchen where he not only had to walk unaided but also to carry and move items around. The walking programme also included increasing his range of walking in that he was able to walk through the grounds to the industrial therapy unit, and so that he could eventually walk to nearby shops, half a mile away, do his shopping and walk back (see Chapter 4). In total the walking programme lasted for 14 months.

CASE REPORT THREE

I.D. fell off his bicycle and sustained a severe head injury at the age of 13. He was unconscious for several months following the accident. There was a previous history of behaviour problems, including being uncooperative and disruptive, and he was in a remedial group at school. Two years after his accident I.D. was still totally dependent for all his needs, fed by nasogastric tube and registered as totally blind. He was also aphonic.

In 1982 he returned home in a wheelchair; he was able to dress himself, transfer from his wheelchair and crawl. Over the following two years the home situation broke down completely.

Following admission and during assessment I.D. was found to have increased muscle tone in all four limbs. He was unable to isolate movements in his right wrist and hand, and the right foot and ankle. All four limbs were poorly coordinated, particularly the right arm. Joint position sense was impaired in the toes. He could move fairly well from one position to another in lying, sitting and kneeling and was able to achieve a high kneeling position. He was unable to stand up unaided or walk. Sitting was also a problem in that I.D. usually flexed at the waist, and because of a flexion deformity at the junction of the cervical and thoracic spines he had to rotate his head to the side in order to see anything. This poor posture had many further implications. Breathing and swallowing were both difficult, and this was exacerbated by poor posture. The same was true of his visual problems, and he also found communication difficult with limited eye-contact.

Walking was just possible using a ladder-back frame and two people supporting him. Trunk control was poor and I.D. flexed to the left side. His head and neck were flexed and his head rotated to the left. He had no heel-strike on either side and

Figure 5.2: Improvement in the percentage of walking with correct head posture using mercury switch headband to provide contingent music reinforcement

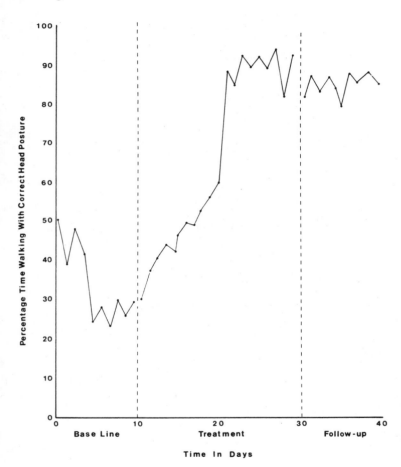

ankle stability was extremely poor on both sides, and both feet were everted. He had very little hip extension whilst walking.

Physiotherapy sessions were initially aimed at improving I.D.'s posture in sitting and standing, and in joint speech/ physiotherapy sessions work was done on the control of breathing and swallowing. Head control, balance and gait were also areas worked on. I.D. made good progress in all of these

111

areas, particularly balance and gait. His sitting and standing balance improved with better head control than he had shown previously.

I.D. started a walking programme. He was able to walk short distances using just a rollator for support and a series of prompts designed to encourage a more correct and rhythmic walking pattern. The prompts consisted of:

(1) 'Push' — prompting him to push his frame a short distance forward.
(2) 'Step' — to take one step.
(3) 'Stretch' — this prompted him to stand up straight, and hold his head up with his mouth closed.

This programme worked well, but it was noticed that I.D. only ever stood up correctly following a prompt of 'stretch', so therefore collaboration with psychologists led to the development of a programme to overcome the problem. Using the fact that I.D. found music very rewarding a procedure was instituted whereby I.D. wore a headband during sessions. The headband was fitted with a mercury switch such that when I.D.'s head was correctly positioned the switch completed a circuit and operated a portable cassette player containing a tape of I.D.'s favourite music. Thus, the correct positioning of the head produced immediate reinforcement of the desired behaviour. Figure 5.2 demonstrates the effectiveness of this procedure. Even following the cessation of music reinforcement it was found that the appropriate head posture continued above the baseline level, possibly because I.D. gained the reinforcement of attention and eye-contact.

CASE REPORT FOUR

D.C. suffered a severe head injury at the age of 28 when he was involved in a road traffic accident. Following the accident he was unconscious for 13 days and post-traumatic amnesia lasted for several months. Previous attempts at rehabilitation had been unsuccessful.

Initial assessment revealed his principal problems as lack of drive and motivation, aggressive outbursts, poor attention to task, incontinence, immobility due to a severe spastic hemiplegia with sensory inattention. He was unable to walk and had poor and often dangerous wheelchair control. Transferring was

Table 5.1

1. Position wheelchair with left side alongside and close to a chair
2. Apply the brakes
3. Put feet in a good position; flat and apart
4. Clasp hands together with elbows stretched
5. Lean forwards
6. Stand up
7. Turn to the left
8. Check chair is behind by looking and feeling
9. Lean forwards
10. Sit down

Figure 5.3: Improvement in transferring from wheelchair to chair using a shaping procedure and contingent reinforcement (taken from Wood, 1984)

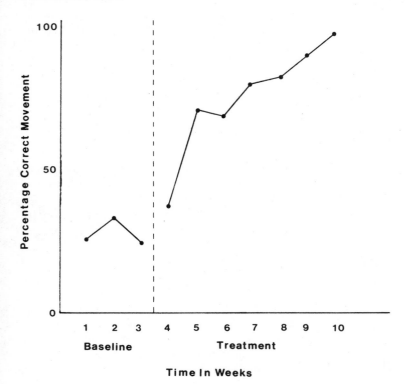

also a problem in that he literally threw himself from chair to chair with little regard for his own or anyone else's safety.

Many different aspects of his physical rehabilitation were covered, but one particular problem was that of transferring. Baseline measures were completed and a transfer programme implemented, aimed at improving his skill and performance in transferring (Goodman-Smith and Turnbull, 1983). It was hoped that this would increase his awareness and effective use of his left side.

The transfer programme consisted of ten units (see Table 5.1). The number of words used in each instruction were kept to a minimum to aid clear understanding. For example in prompt '3' the command given was 'Feet flat and apart', and in '4', it was 'Clasp hands, stretch elbows'.

Each unit in the programme which was achieved was immediately rewarded with a small sweet and plenty of congratulation and praise. The programme was repeated five times each day (see Figure 5.3).

During baseline recordings the proportion of correct movements completed in the transfer programme was 26 per cent. During the course of the programme, which continued for six months, this increased from 40 to 90 per cent. At this stage D.C. was five years post-accident. He eventually went on to walk unaided.

CONCLUSION

The attentional and cognitive problems associated with severe brain injury present a major challenge to physiotherapists working in this area. Traditional forms of physiotherapy, it is argued, must give way to techniques that are functionally based. The task of the physiotherapist is to help brain-injured people to relearn new skills. However, attentional and cognitive deficits severely decrease learning ability and therefore to set the task in a functional or lifelike setting is to increase the chances of satisfactory outcome.

The need for close interdisciplinary liaison is demonstrated, in order to increase the functional relevance of tasks to be relearned, and of course this requires the physiotherapist to become more aware of learning processes, and how they can be disrupted. This is exemplified by the breaking down of tasks into units that are relevant to the patient. For the brain-injured person, physiotherapy can only produce meaningful change by facilitating the relearning of tasks that are likely to be relevant to the patient in the future.

6

Treating Communication Disorders in the Brain-injured Adult

Carmella Mazzella-Gordon and Kelley L. Wicks

Effective communication depends not only on the correct articulation of words; it also demands a sophisticated system of socially appropriate verbal and non-verbal behaviours which together enable a person to function in society. Following brain injury the complex processes underlying normal communication may be disturbed. Damage may be diffuse and disrupt widely separate areas of brain tissue — leading to, at one extreme, severely disordered linguistic ability, and at the other, subclinical linguistic disorders (Sarno, 1984).

Once the patient emerges from coma the therapist will begin to assess how much the patient can understand and how the patient can best communicate. Differential diagnosis delineates the various factors involved in the breakdown of speech and language skills. The therapist must continually educate and counsel patient and family about communicative difficulties. An alternative means of communication may have to be established in order to allow patients to express needs; for example 'yes/no' systems and word charts or alphabet boards. Prolonged intubation may result in drooling and difficulties with swallowing, which must also be assessed and treated.

Therapeutic intervention can be divided into four areas:

(1) *Evaluation*: assessment of specific speech and language skills and of functional communicative abilities;
(2) *Specific skills training*: carrying out structured therapy programmes to deal with specific areas of deficit;
(3) *Functional treatment*: helping the patient to communicate effectively in a variety of real-world situations;

(4) *Education and counselling*: educating the patient, family and staff about the patient's communicative problems and current treatment programmes.

EVALUATION

A formal speech and language evaluation is required for all brain-injured patients even when language deficits are not immediately apparent. Sarno (1984) reports that over a third of all closed-head injury patients with a history of coma have hidden linguistic deficits. The evaluation should include auto-biographical information, observations and an oral interview as well as standardised testing. Evaluation allows differential diagnosis and helps to establish a baseline of performance.

Informal assessment

Prior to administering formal tests the patient should be assessed informally. This assessment consists of observing the patient as he or she enters the room, taking note of level of awareness, initiation and responsiveness. In initial convers-ations the speech therapist can check for temporal and spatial orientation, and orientation to person. The speech therapist should observe for gross signs of dysarthria, apraxia, aphasia, non-verbal communicative ability, and receptive problems. The patient's apparent motivation to communicate should also be noted. The results of this interview assist the therapist in selecting the most appropriate formal tests.

Formal assessment

A variety of formal assessments may be used to discern the patient's strengths and weaknesses. Therapists should select tests which meet their needs in terms of the time required for test presentation and the type of results derived. Areas the speech therapist may wish to assess include dysphasic disorders, motor speech disorders, functional communication in real-world settings, cognitive skills and academic skills. Whether the latter two categories are assessed by the speech therapist depends on local practice, and these will not be discussed further here.

Among tests of dysphasic disorders the Boston Diagnostic Aphasia Examination (BDAE) (Goodglass and Kaplan, 1972) provides tools for identifying expressive language and auditory comprehension disorders. Verbal responses are analysed for completeness, appropriateness, syntactical correctness and complexity. Complete administration of the BDAE is lengthy and should be performed over a number of days. The BDAE is appropriate for all except the highest functioning patients who might have subtle deficits. The Western Aphasia Battery (WAB) (Kertesz, 1982) was designed to evaluate content, fluency, auditory comprehension, repetition, and naming as well as reading, writing and calculation. The oral portion of the test can be administered in an hour. Test results render an 'aphasia quotient' (AQ) from the oral portion of the test and a 'cortical quotient' (CQ) from the non-verbal scores. The WAB allows classification of patients' language according to type of aphasia (Kertesz and Poole, 1974). The Minnesota Test for the Differential Diagnosis of Aphasia (MTDDA) (Schuell, 1963) tests language performance in the brain-injured in the areas of auditory skills, visual and reading skills, speech/language skills, visuomotor and writing skills and numerical relations and arithmetic processes. The MTDDA renders five diagnostic categories which correlate with neurological findings and which indicate likely prognosis. While it yields considerable information it is difficult to use and may be time-consuming.

For obvious reasons it is difficult to develop a standardised test for motor speech. *Motor Speech Disorders* (Darley *et al.*, 1975), however, provides a thorough description of (1) assessment of speech mechanisms during non-speech activities, (2) assessment of motor speech, (3) assessment of motor speech for determination of dyspraxia of speech. The authors also provide a detailed discussion of the therapeutic interventions for motor speech disorders.

Some clients will retain a remarkable ability to communicate despite severe dysphasic disorder. The Functional Communication Profile devised by Taylor-Sarno (1965) provides an early example of a test of communication skills in real-life settings. A more complete and now more widely used evaluation is the Communicative Abilities of Daily Living (CADL) (Holland, 1980). This test includes categories such as estimating and calculating time, using social conventions and appreciating humour.

No single test is likely to cover all areas of relevance, and the therapist will need to develop a test battery which can be used depending on need. These brief descriptions of some of the many available tests illustrate areas to be assessed, and point to some of the issues relevant to test selection.

Factors to be considered in evaluation

During the evaluation process the speech therapist should consider the patient in his total environmental context. Attitudes of family members and associates should be considered, as well as those of the patient. For example the family may not agree that communicative independence is necessary. It is important to determine the patient's need for speech and to obtain a clear picture of his everyday activities (Johnson *et al.*, 1963).

A wide range of factors may affect speech production. Not only may mood disorders affect speech, medication administered to the head-injured patient for control of epilepsy, aggression or affective disturbance may produce dysarthria and/or reduced language function. Even after discontinuation of medication it may take weeks or months for some side-effects to disappear. Disorders of attention can also affect all aspects of speech and language. The patient may be distractible, appear confused, or demonstrate poor concentration (Goldenson *et al.*, 1978) resulting in hesitant speech, inappropriate responses, circumlocutions, or the need for repetition. The patient may lose track of what has been asked, what he is saying or the point he wanted to make. Within the structured test environment the patient may focus attention and perform well on individual items. The therapist must observe the patient outside the structured testing environment to determine if the patient can sustain attention given competing stimuli. For example, the patient may be unable to participate in a conversation at mealtime or other group settings.

SPECIFIC SKILLS TRAINING

Dysphasia

Dysphasia may be defined as a disturbance of the complex process of comprehending and formulating verbal messages that results from acquired disease of the central nervous system. Often, dysphasic patients have difficulty with both understanding language (receptive disturbances) and producing language in written, oral, or gestural form (expressive disturbances). Moreover, in dysphasia, the various forms of language processing, e.g. listening, speaking and writing, can be disturbed to different degrees.

It is often difficult to evaluate receptive disorders because the therapist must separate environmental clues from auditory input. Often the patient will respond to environmental clues, which can give speakers the impression that the patient can understand more of the spoken component of the message than is the case. Moreover the patient may not communicate to the speaker any difficulty understanding the spoken message.

In the early stages of treatment information should be presented to more than one sensory system (Hawley, 1984). Attempts to treat the disorder should begin at or below the patient's level in order to allow success early in therapy. Typically patients improve in a range of language skills so that as auditory comprehension increases, word-finding errors decrease, patients begin to talk in longer, better-formulated responses, and reading, writing and arithmetic also improve (Schuell, 1974). A typical programme of auditory stimulation involving increasingly complex tasks is provided in Table 6.1. With patients who are functioning at a higher level, more complex tasks should be attempted, such as comprehension of lengthier passages requiring sustained attention, integration, inference and drawing conclusions; both spoken and written materials should be used. Tasks where deficits may be apparent in some higher-functioning patients include recall of the sequence of information, recall of details, and being able to summarise.

The highest level of comprehension is the ability to make a judgement about what has been heard or read. In order to make a judgement one must first have heard the information, interpreted it, and then compared it to values and previously

Table 6.1: Auditory comprehension tasks

Auditory recognition of common words
Discrimination of paired words
Auditory recognition of named letters
Identification of words named in pictures
Following one- to three-step directions
Understanding yes/no questions
Understanding a paragraph
Repeat digits
Repeat sentences

acquired knowledge. Head-injured patients often accomplish literal comprehension tasks because these tasks require only concrete thinking. Due to cognitive deficits some patients may have difficulty with interpretive comprehension tasks. For example patient J.A. was recovering well after a severe head injury six months previously. He had moderate language impairment but he was able to live independently. He was attending as an outpatient for assessment prior to returning to work as a master mechanic. On assessment it was discovered that J.A. had severe difficulty in understanding complex verbal and written instructions. So while he could follow three- or four-step verbal commands with little apparent difficulty, he had great difficulty in understanding written instructions, a factor which would be significant in his employment. In this case treatment involved convincing J.A. that reading was indeed an area of difficulty. He was then taught compensatory techniques which he could use at work such as reviewing instructions with a co-worker.

Expressive difficulties

The patient with expressive language deficits has difficulty in remembering and using specific words. Word-finding difficulties are exhibited through delays in production, use of associations and descriptions, and the use of non-specific words, e.g. 'thing'. Sentence formulation strategies are disordered and consequently utterances violate syntactic rules. The patient's language will be marked by an abundance of starters, fillers, circumlocutions, indefinite references and word substitutions. The patient may also perseveratively repeat words, phrases or clauses and the patient's language may have an 'empty' quality.

Typically therapeutic interventions for mild to moderate expressive language deficits may include both verbal and reading tasks, and a selection of these are shown in Table 6.2.

Table 6.2: Tasks used in the treatment of patients with expressive language deficits

Verbal tasks
    word repetition
    phrase repetition
    automatic speech
    sentence completion
    answering simple questions
    providing biographical information
    expressing ideas
    producing sentences given words
    defining words
    describing pictures
    confrontation naming
    retelling paragraphs

Reading tasks
    matching words to pictures
    matching printed to spoken words
    responding to printed yes/no questions
    paragraphs of increasing length
    reading words, sentences and paragraphs in unison
    independent oral reading of words, sentences and paragraphs

Writing tasks
    copying designs
    writing numbers
    reproducing designs from memory
    reproducing letters
    written spelling
    oral spelling
    writing sentences to dictation

Facilitative techniques may also be used. One such technique is called deblocking (LaPointe, 1978). Deblocking consists of using intact language modes (e.g. visual perception) to facilitate the use of modes that are functioning at less than optimum levels (e.g. auditory processing). The speech therapist attempts to maximise residual language skills by the use of language channels that are more functional. Other methods include the compensatory approach which, for example, encourages patients to ask for repetition if they need it (some of these methods are briefly reviewed by Kertesz, 1985). In general terms the primary form of therapy for dysphasia is exposing patients to language and encouraging the development of individualised strategies.

Dyspraxia

Dyspraxia is a disturbance in the programming of voluntary muscle control without paralysis or weakness (Emerick and Hatton, 1974). Dyspraxia can be exhibited in the oral musculature (oral dyspraxia), in motor activities (limb dyspraxia), or in speech production (verbal dyspraxia). Patients with verbal dyspraxia have lost the automaticity of correct sound, syllable and word sequencing. Each type of dyspraxia may occur independently, or they may coexist.

Rosenbeck *et al.* (1973) assembled an eight-step task continuum to improve patients' capacity for volitional–purposeful communication. In order to move from one step to the next a patient is required to achieve 80 per cent accuracy over 20 consecutive responses. Deal and Florance (1978) revised the Rosenbeck *et al.* (1973) eight-step continuum so that patients had only to drill steps one to four using a more rigid criterion of accuracy. In this programme the therapist and patient establish ten sentences which comprise a natural conversational exchange in a familiar setting, such as 'breakfast time'. The four steps are: (1) simultaneous production, (2) the patient produces the sentence while the clinician mouths the sentence, (3) one imitation, (4) three consecutive imitations (Deal and Florance, 1978).

Dysarthria

Dysarthria is a collective name for a group of related speech disorders that are due to disturbances in muscular control of the speech mechanism resulting from impairment of any of the basic motor processes involved in the execution of speech (Darley *et al.*, 1975). Dysarthria is characterised by distorted articulation, phonation or resonance. Dysarthrias are generally categorised into types: flaccid dysarthria, spastic dysarthria, mixed flaccid–spastic dysarthria, hypokinetic (Parkinsonian)

123

dysarthria, hyperkinetic dysarthria and ataxic dysarthria. Speech production in the dysarthric patient may be weak, hypernasal and slurred, and may have a disturbed rate or volume. Patients may display several deviant speech characteristics at once.

A range of treatment methods for the dysarthrias are reported in *Dysarthria and Apraxia* (Perkins, 1983). Aten (1983) recommends isolating a critical dimension of speech and focusing initially on eliminating the negative aspects of that characteristic. Repetition of single words, phrases and sentences may be effective in improving performance. As early as possible, the patient should be trained to monitor the quality and intelligibility of his speech. Aten further notes that medical or prosthetic interventions (such as palatal lifts) should be considered before intensive speech therapy is begun (Aten, 1983). Familiar and practically useful material should be practised over and over again. Tape recording may be used to provide feedback and improve accuracy.

FUNCTIONAL TREATMENT

Functional communication, and not necessarily a return to premorbid language levels, is the primary goal of therapy (LaPointe, 1978). Due to the head-injured patient's difficulties with abstract thinking, and using a skill learned in one situation in another situation, a functional approach is essential. Whenever possible the speech therapist should design therapy tasks to incorporate activities which the patient will need to perform after he leaves the treatment facility. Examples of appropriate therapy tasks depend on the likely functional level of the patient, but may include asking to go to the toilet, asking for help or asking for something to be passed at table to obtaining information in the community, going through the process of enrolling in classes, using public transportation, filling out job applications, telephone use, word processing, proof-reading, summarising, comprehension of recipes, following complex or incomplete directions, balancing a cheque book, organising personal correspondence and knowledge and practice of response to emergency situations. Tasks selected for therapy should be consistent with patients' past and present interests, be realistic and achievable given the existing deficits and meet the patient's needs for communication.

Only by watching the patient engage in the task will the therapist develop an adequate understanding of all components of the situation with which the patient will be faced. Initially the therapist needs to provide prompts to ensure adequate performance. Appropriate, but not excessive, cues or facilitators are essential. The therapist must continually reassess the patient's performance, and adjust or eliminate cues when necessary.

A range of adaptive equipment may help the individual with communication deficits. These aids can range from a portable typewriter, display printer or computer, to a simple communication or alphabet board. Non-verbal patients may have severe language impairments that prevent their use of an aid, but this should not be assumed, and a reasonable training trial of at least two weeks should be allowed. Important considerations in designing a communication board are ease of use to the client (Wu and Voda, 1985) and relevance to the patient's daily activities. The patient needs to be trained to use the board in the functional settings of daily life, and the speech therapist should train other staff in how to interact with the patient using the board (Calculator and Luchko, 1983; Coleman et al., 1980).

For head-injured patients practice in the type of environment they are actually likely to encounter is indicated. A patient's increased level of anxiety in new situations may lead to impulsive reactions. Exposure to these situations may lead to a great increase in level of performance due to reduced anxiety. T.K.'s treatment provides an example of frequent practice of real-world tasks increasing independence. T.K. was a 17-year-old male who sustained a severe head injury from a fall. Duration of coma was in excess of two weeks, and treatment occurred when T.K. was two years post-injury. T.K. had severe word-finding difficulties and moderate to severe verbal apraxia, as well as moderate auditory comprehension difficulties. His functional level of performance at home and in the residential setting was surprisingly good, but on a number of occasions he was noted to be incapable of ordering items when out in shops and restaurants. Beginning on a sessional basis work was begun to prepare for a trip to a local coffee house. The patient had to determine what he would like to order, how much money to take, and the fact that, due to his use of a walker, the patient would have to ask one of the employees to carry his coffee to a table for him. The speech therapist wrote a brief 'script' which covered the necessary three or four conversational exchanges. Intensive practice continued over a week with various staff members. The speech therapist provided visual and contextual cues, such as standing behind a desk to simulate the counter, speaking quickly, and asking the patient to repeat when his volume was low or articulation was not easily intelligible.

Next the speech therapist accompanied T.K. to the coffee house. T.K. independently ordered and paid for the coffee, without assistance from the therapist. However, after T.K. had paid, the salesperson moved to the next customer. Although T.K. wanted his coffee to be carried to a table he did nothing to gain the attention of the salesperson, and the speech therapist had to intervene to indicate that the patient had another request. The patient was then easily able to complete his communication and get himself, and his coffee, to a table. T.K. was pleased and enthusiastic about his successful interaction outside of the sheltered transitional living centre. T.K. indicated that he would like to order a dessert, as well as coffee, the next time. Practice followed the same routine. On returning to the coffee shop, T.K. ordered his items and requested assistance to the table with no intervention by the speech therapist. This level of performance was maintained at three-month follow-up and was being used in novel settings.

In some patients straightforward practice will not meet all of the patient's needs and a behavioural approach is indicated. Ince (1973) was able to improve the word-finding ability of an aphasic man, using verbal reinforcement and feedback of results. Goodkin (1966) used behavioural methods with an aphasic woman who was three years post-injury. She would switch rapidly from one subject to another, and her answers to questions were generally inappropriate. Verbal and tangible reinforcement produced a significant improvement in ability to respond appropriately. A wide range of behavioural approaches have been used with success in the brain-damaged population (Goodkin, 1969). Wood and Eames (1981) report work with a patient who had made a good (but not perfect) physical and intellectual recovery but her reintegration into the outside world was marred by her production of continuous, repetitive and extremely rapid themes, most of which were socially inappropriate. Treatment involved a number of elements: specific speech therapy to establish control over speech production; sessional cognitive overlearning of what was appropriate and a time-out-on-the-spot procedure. The authors report an impressive reduction in the unacceptable aspects of her speech production.

An important use for behavioural methods by the speech therapist can be helping patients to use skills that have been acquired in speech therapy sessions in their daily lives when this is proving problematic. Table 6.3 gives an example of a type of programme that may be devised to help patients overcome this problem.

Table 6.3: An example of a token reinforcement programme to help a patient establish good speech outside speech therapy sessions

Problem   Rapid, poorly articulated, and mumbled speech and frequently incomprehensible speech production

Criterion   To be acceptable speech should be loud enough and produced slowly enough that it is possible to understand every word that is said, the first time that it is said.

Tokens   Each statement that meets this criterion earns a token and verbal praise (i.e. 'that was very clear and slow; well done!'). Statements which do not meet this criterion are to be timed out on the spot (TOOTSed), if a repeat attempt is clear it should be responded to but no token given. Tokens are not given for single-word utterances.

Reinforcement   All tokens to be handed in at 5 o'clock; 50 tokens in one day leads to a T-bone steak dinner.

Recording   Record token earnings on sheet provided. Programme to be reviewed in two weeks from date of commencement.

EDUCATION AND COUNSELLING

The discrepancy between real and apparent ability has practical consequences for all aspects of rehabilitation, can be easily overlooked, and may lead to unrealistic expectations, resulting in feelings of helplessness and frustration. The speech therapist should ensure that all those therapeutically involved with a patient who has speech or language impairment understand the limitations these disorders may impose. For example an individual with receptive difficulties may be unable to follow simple and/or complex commands. Failure to answer questions or monosyllabic responses may be due to expressive language difficulties rather than due to an unwillingness to speak. An apparently curt remark may have been an attempt at a joke, but lack of intonation masks the intention. Someone who can respond to greetings and shows no difficulty with simple social exchange may have severe difficulties in comprehension and expression. Educating the family about the disability, and enlisting their participation in a programme of rehabilitation, is a major responsibility of rehabilitation personnel.

Many patients who make an otherwise good recovery will retain subtle language deficits. These may persist and emerge again in later life. Changing circumstances — perhaps a new line of study, a new job, or a promotion — place different and unexpected demands upon language processing and expression. Some patients may learn to avoid situations which demonstrate their areas of deficit. Some learn to compensate and to use adaptive strategies to reduce the consequences of their problems. Some do not spontaneously acquire compensatory strategies, and need assistance in developing adaptive and efficient techniques for compensation. Communication deficits may continue to have a negative influence on the quality of interpersonal relationships.

Prolonged institutionalisation can have a very damaging effect on the long-term recovery of the patient. The tendency of others not to demand speech of the language-disordered patient may lead to further functional incapacity. Some speech or language patterns may have become habitual, so that even though a patient's ability might have improved the performance is still functionally disordered (see Chapter 1). Similarly, some patterns may have been reinforced inadvertently by others: a patient who is perfectly capable of asking for a light for a cigarette may gain instant response to a gesture and therefore learns he never has to ask. Both family and staff should be aware of receptive language difficulties and the patient's ability to compensate for them by, for example, relying on gestural cues. Family and staff may frequently report that 'He understands everything we say', but removal of situational cues demonstrates severe deficits. Conversely observers may magnify the patient's disabilities and come to believe the patient is more handicapped than he really is, and may unnecessarily restrict the quality and quantity of their speech. Wherever language difficulties are present supportive therapy from a group of fellow-patients can be beneficial in reducing the isolation of the disabled, giving them a different perspective on their condition, and can discover areas of intactness by falling back on old and trusted social conventions.

Lack of insight into problems may lead to inappropriate speech with the patient failing to regulate output. Patients who are overconscious of problems may withdraw from contact or devise strategies to cope, which could add to the communication problem. An example of this is T.K. (previously described) with severe expressive aphasia, who spoke very quietly so he would be less embarrassed if he made a mistake, but took this to such an extreme that he could not be heard at all. Even when good speech and language ability is preserved, deviation from normal social behaviour will high-light the fact that something is 'wrong' with the patient, e.g. inappropriate posture, facial expression, gesture, intonation, invasion of personal space, eye-contact, misuse of conversational rules and turn-taking. Sharing information with other staff may highlight any further discrepancies in performance. Work may need to be taken into these domains to increase the patient's social skills and hence social acceptability.

The speech therapist can both directly and indirectly assist in the rehabilitation of communication skills, by considering communication in a functional sense and applying skills outside the traditional clinical setting.

7

Conductive Education and Motor Learning

Gordon Muir Giles and Ann Gent

Brain-injured adults can display a vast range of physical deficits. Unfortunately their concurrent cognitive problems often limit their ability to overcome their physical dysfunction. Patients may have disorders of memory, attention and perception. They may also have disorders of drive and behaviour which make it difficult to establish and maintain participation in therapy. The therapist often spends more time trying to induce the patient to cooperate than in actually providing therapy (Gent and Giles, 1986). Memory problems often mean that the patient has no recollection of ever having had therapy, let alone the content of the individual sessions.

Therapy for motor disorders can be approached from a number of perspectives including the neurodevelopmental (Bobath, 1978) and the biomechanical (Nasher and McCollum, 1985). Discussions of therapy typically ignore learning in general, and motor learning in particular. By examining those factors which affect learning it should be possible to describe an intervention strategy which maximises the individual's chances for learning. The individual with neurological disorders following brain injury has a body which no longer functions in the way it used to. The rules which governed what constitutes effective motor output have changed, and for the patient to function after injury new rules must be learned. In this chapter we will examine some of the main theories which underlie current thinking on motor learning. These theories involve attempts to explain how movements are planned, selected and remembered, and how they are controlled as they are being executed, and can be used to help therapists design the most appropriate type of intervention. We will then describe conductive education, suggesting that it be used as a model of rehabilitation after brain injury. For a general review of conductive education, see Cottam and Sutton (1985).

WHY USE CONDUCTIVE EDUCATION?

Conductive education provides many of the factors shown to be relevant to learning motor control described in the first part of this chapter:

(1) it is goal-directed and achievement-oriented,
(2) it teaches needed functional skills,
(3) it encourages repeated practice,
(4) it provides organisation and 'labels' to help patients retain sequences,
(5) it encourages the patient's modelling,
(6) it is particularly suited for patients with attentional and memory deficits,
(7) it helps teach patients methods to control their inappropriate movements.

Conductive education provides a model of rehabilitation because it incorporates many of the factors which, when used individually, have been shown to increase the rate of learning or the period of retention of motor tasks. These factors are discussed with regard to feedback and motor learning, attentional variables and motor learning, practice, other factors affecting motor learning and cognitive factors. As well as being relevant to the individual components of conductive education this discussion will inform therapists the way current research would suggest they structure their treatment sessions. Many of the principles described later in this chapter derive from, or make reference to, theories of motor learning; however these theories do not make easy reading and the reader with less interest in this area is encouraged to proceed directly to the section on feedback and motor learning.

THEORIES OF MOTOR LEARNING

Adams's (1971, 1976) closed-loop theory of motor learning proposed the existence of a self-regulatory feedback system to account for motor control. The two essential components of this theory are the perceptual trace and the memory trace. According to this theory the memory trace is a stored set of instructions responsible for the initial selection and direction of movement, while the perceptual trace is a stored version of the perceptual information fed back during the actual movement. The perceptual trace is responsible for error correction and directing the body during the actual movement. The process of learning a movement is the development of a perceptual trace which is dependent on feedback and error correction (Adams, 1977). The greater the amount of feedback available the stronger the perceptual trace. Accepting the closed-loop theoretical framework implies that continuous sensory feedback is necessary for motor control, but recent evidence has suggested that this is not the case (Bizzi and Polit, 1979; Schmidt, 1982; Taub and Berman, 1968).

It has been suggested that ballistic movements may be the result of a central control without continuous feedback. Hammering a nail, or typing by an experienced typist, are examples of movements which may be too rapid to allow use to be made of feedback during the execution of the action. This 'open-loop' theory (Schmidt, 1975, 1976) suggests that control of movement is possible because a motor programme exists which contains all the necessary information to regulate a movement without reference to continuous feedback. Indeed extremely well-rehearsed patterns of movement appear to be disrupted by attempts to attend to them (Reason, 1979). Some of the strongest evidence for the existence of motor programmes comes from analysis of highly overlearned activities such as walking and running in experienced runners (Shapiro *et al.*, 1981), typing (Terzuolo and Viviani, 1979) and writing (Merton, 1972).

Both open- and closed-loop theories have been subject to criticism (see Mulder and Hulstijn, 1984, for a discussion). A more parsimonious explanation has been offered by Schmidt in the form of 'schema' theory, which is an attempt to overcome some of the problems of open-loop theory by reducing the amount of information accommodated in each motor programme (Schmidt, 1975, 1976; Mulder and Hulstijn, 1984). In this theory the schema is an abstract memory construct which governs a motor act. The schema is formed by the attempt to execute a particular motor act, and is built up from what is learned from the various experiences of the action. An individual does not retain a memory of each time a movement is performed, but does retain a generalised memory which has been abstracted from the various experiences. Schmidt suggests that the motor programme is only a general plan, and that it includes within it latitude to accommodate the demands of individual circumstances. So force, direction, speed and other factors might be varied within an individual schema with the individual being assumed to modify the programme in response to circumstance. An alternative notion has been to look at motor performance as 'action' (Turvey, 1977; Reed, 1982; Stelmach and Diggles, 1982). The highest level in action theory is the action plan which is specific in terms of outcome but not in terms of the method of achieving it, underlying the fact that humans are able to use different methods to achieve the same end. For example an individual may put on a pair of shoes by bending down to the ground, resting his foot on a chair, or may sit in a chair and cross his legs. The notion is heterarchical (as opposed to hierarchical) because there is no one source of a motor programme; control is distributed across various levels which interact to fulfil the action plan (Turvey, 1977). Central to action theories are not motor systems or motor output but function. The belief which underlies this is that behaviour may be neurologically and psychologically organised in terms of function. This concept is similar to older Russian notions of functional systems where an invariant aim is achieved by variable mechanisms and achieving the (invariant) goal (Luria, 1973). Postures and movements are examined in the larger framework of actions and context. The elements of a task performance, it is suggested, are governed at different levels (spinal cord, brainstem, cerebellum, cerebrum) but the action of these systems must be coordinated and directed towards a goal (Gibson, 1966; Reed, 1982).

Action theory represented by Gibson, Reed and others (Gibson, 1966; Reed, 1982; Turvey, 1977) stand apart from the mainstream of thinking in regard to how motor behaviour is governed. Consensus seems to support the notion of a central-ised motor programme (which specifies some aspects of movement but not others) and which is modified when possible by feedback. So, for example, throwing darts or hammering a nail are thought of as pre-programmed movements not adjusted by ongoing feedback, while slower movements do seem to be influenced by continuous feedback. Automatic movements — such as walking and postural adjustments — also seem to rely on motor programmes. These 'motor primitives' may originate in the basal ganglia and be refined in execution by the cerebellum (Stein, 1985).

FEEDBACK AND MOTOR LEARNING

With the exception of practice, feedback is probably the most important single factor to be considered in motor learning (Winstein, 1987). Feedback can be of two kinds: internal or external. Internal feedback includes not only information coming from specialised receptors in muscles, joints, tendons and the skin, but also from vision (Gibson, 1966). Internal feedback is extremely impoitant, but not essential, for the learning of some movements. Gross movements such as walking and simple reaching may not require continual feedback for their execution (Bach-y-Rita et al., 1987). Other tasks, such as sustained grasp, may require continuous feedback. Therapists will often attempt to direct the patient's attention to intrinsic feedback by, for example, asking the patient about sensations in an attempt to help the patient learn what sitting upright feels like. External feedback refers to feedback which does not necessarily arise as a result of movement and is provided by an external source. The possible modes of presentation of external feedback are numerous. They may be auditory (non-verbal as in beeps and buzzes), lines on a visual display, lights, or as a switching mechanism operating a computer, a radio or other appliance (case report 3, Chapter 5, may be interpreted as an example of this). All of these methods have meaning to the learner and are methods of giving him or her more information than would otherwise be available. More frequently used is verbal feedback. External feedback, whatever its mode of presentation, can be provided in two forms: knowledge of results (sometimes called learning feedback) and knowledge of performance (sometimes called action feedback). Knowledge of results (KR) is defined as information about the consequences of an action or series of actions (Salmoni *et al.*, 1984). KR may be particularly important where there is limited sensory feedback. Although in some cases KR may be obvious (e.g. an individual will know if in attempting to transfer from a bed to a wheelchair he falls); in other cases it may not be (e.g. the patient may be unable to determine when an upright posture has been achieved).

Another type of external feedback is knowledge of performance (KP). Whereas KR is information about the end-result of a movement, KP is information about the means to the end, i.e. the movement pattern used. The therapist can provide information not only about the goal but also about the attempted method. Winstein (1987) suggests that KP is more appropriate for use in the therapeutic setting because a patient may know that he failed to successfully perform a task, but may not be aware of the factors which underlie the failure and because there are often several components to the desired movement outcome. Patients can only improve their performance if they know where it broke down. For example a patient may be aware of difficulties in drinking from a cup (KR), but not be aware that performance is poor because of a failure to keep his wrist extended (KP).

There is clear evidence that learning is enhanced by feedback (Mulder and Hulstijn, 1984). In the brain-injured patient feedback is often distorted or in some cases absent. Patients may have great difficulty in attending to the significant aspects of their environments. It may be that providing adequate external feedback may help the patient compensate for these deficits. External feedback such as verbal cueing can provide additional information and thereby aid performance. If the movement is thought to be in accord with the closed-loop model, then feedback during performance may be helpful. If the movement is fast, and thought to approximate the open-loop model, then feedback of KR and KP can be used to help improve inter-trial performance. In both cases subjects can use feedback in error correction. The more types of feedback which are available, the greater the learning. Ensuring that some degree of success is achieved by patients is likely to encourage further effort, while continual experience of failure will reduce the amount of effort the subject expends (Brame, 1979).

The optimum amount of KR is not known; too frequent use of KR could increase performance but decrease learning and patients may become dependent on feedback. The most effective schedule of feedback is not known, and needs to be assessed by the therapist. In early learning an arbitrary figure of 50 per cent feedback may be appropriate, and the degree of feedback reduced as mastery is attained. Research is needed with the brain-injured in order to establish the factors which determine the optimum feedback ratio.

ATTENTIONAL VARIABLES AND MOTOR LEARNING

Another important consideration in planning rehabilitation programmes is the patient's ability to attend to the significant aspects of what is being taught, a particular problem for the brain-injured. Shiffrin and Schneider (1977) have discussed attention in terms of automatic versus control processing. Prior to injury the patient could perform a large number of activities without paying attention to them; performance was largely automatic. For example most people walk without directing any conscious attention to the location of their feet or consciously controlling their posture. After injury if the patient is to attempt to perform an action such as sitting upright active attention must be directed towards the task. This conscious process is both frustrating and tiring, but is required if automatic processing is to develop (Schneider et al., 1984). There is also a limit to the number of processes that can be attended to at any one time. Schneider and Shiffrin describe this limitation as a divided attentional deficit (DAD). Here too much information is coming in for the individual to process in the time available. For example at certain stages of rehabilitation a patient may be able to walk independently unless someone walks across his visual field or says 'good morning', whereupon the patient falls over. This constitutes a DAD because the patient has insufficient attentional capacity to walk and to attend to anything else. Another way in which performance can be disrupted due to a limitation of attention is described by Schneider and Shiffrin as a focused attentional deficit (FAD). A FAD typically occurs when an unfamiliar response is required to a stimulus which already has a familiar response attached to it. The habitual response is usually the result of previous experience or learning, and may require continuous attention for the subject to suppress this automatic behaviour. So, for example, when trying to help a patient improve his walking pattern the previous poor gait will be produced unless the patient devotes active attention to producing the new one. One of the authors (G.M.G.) saw two patients in a single hospital ward, one very frequently (twice a day), one infrequently (once a week). Despite intending to go to the room of the infrequently seen patient G.M.G. always found himself at the door of the frequently seen patient. The work of Reason (1979) suggests that this kind of 'action not as planned' may be extremely common, and depends to some extent on a Hullian concept of 'habit strength'.

Learning is demonstrated not only by increased competency but also by a reduction in the attentional demands of the task. Fitts (1964) and Fitts and Posner (1967) describe this transition as one from cognitive control, which requires total active attention and in which subjects tend to verbalise each step of the task, through the associative stage and ending in the autonomous stage where the task places only limited attentional demands on the subject. Typically in the autonomous phase the subject loses the ability to verbalise the task (Fitts, 1964). Central to Fitts's notion is the idea that most complex tasks are learned as a number of short simple procedures fitted together. Other variables the therapist should consider in planning treatment are how long the patient can attend to a specific task, the time of day (Watts *et al.*, 1983), the level of distraction in the treatment environment, and so on. One of the aims of therapy is to return the activities that now require effort to the category of automatic processes.

In order for learning to occur sensory information of some type must be available, or there can be no knowledge of error. Where sensory information is thought to be less than optimal various attempts have been made to artificially increase the amount of information available.

Mirrors and video equipment are commonly used to provide visual feedback and to allow patients to monitor their performance. Gibson has demonstrated the crucial role of vision in controlling behaviour (Gibson, 1966, 1979). Reed (1982) cites an experiment conducted by Lishman and Lee (1973) demonstrating that humans walking forward, but exposed to optical information indicating that they are moving backwards, will report that they are moving backwards. Vision plays a crucial role in the maintenance of posture and balance, and is probably mediated via the cerebellum (Stein, 1986). This is particularly true when either vestibular or somatosensory feedback is reduced. Swaying backwards and forwards can be detected by optic flow (if the visual field expands a movement backwards has occurred, if the visual field contracts a movement forward has taken place (Gibson, 1966). The importance of vision in locomotion is demonstrated by the fact that muscle activity used to cushion the effect of stepping down only occurs when the subjects are allowed normal vision. Patients with certain neurological conditions, including Parkinson's disease, who have problems in organising movement, use vision to compensate for their impairments (Stein, 1986; Bach-y-Rita et al., 1987). The addition of visual feedback, not normally available to the subject, has been shown to aid learning in the non-neurologically impaired.

PRACTICE

It seems clear that as movements are repeated changes take place in the way that they are stored and executed, resulting in increased economy of energy expenditure. One way to view this change is to regard the generation of a motor programme as allowing a change to take place from control to automatic processing. A major practical question is how practice can best be used in order to speed learning and maximise retention of what is learned. Much recent work has centred around a prediction derived from schema theory that increased variability of practice on a task will increase transfer of skill to a similar task. Work with children has supported this view fairly consistently (Carson and Wiegand, 1979; Lee et al., 1985) but this is not so in the case of adults where results have been inconsistent (Bird and Rikli, 1983; Catalano and Kleiner, 1984; Husak and Reeve, 1979; Johnson and McCabe, 1982).

Lee et al. (1985) suggest that differences in research design account for the conflicting results. Studies where the variations in task are blocked together (all of one type occurring at once) do not support the prediction from schema theory, whereas random variable practice on a motor task (interchanging first one task then the other in a way that cannot be predicted by the subject) provides strong support for the schema theory prediction (Lee et al., 1985). It has been suggested that when practice is grouped together subjects have some form of memory trace left over from the previous performance which they can use in the repetition of the task. When different tasks are interspersed, however, subjects are unable to use this strategy and must actively attempt to recall and generate the movement pattern *de novo*, leading to a greater ability to generalise. Other workers have examined similar issues from a different perspective. Shea and Morgan (1979) found that in comparing random to blocked practice the blocked repetition facilitated acquisition performance but led to poor retention, while random ordering facilitated retention but was detrimental to acquisition performance. It has been suggested that the differences in performance can, as with generalisation, best be accounted for by suggesting that random practice forces subjects to use more cognitively effortful problem-solving activities.

The discussion above indicates two specific ways to enhance learning. The first is that practice of a task in slightly different ways may result in the subject having a greater ability to generalise the skill to novel situations. For example in training a patient to transfer from his wheelchair varying the heights of the surfaces to be transferred to, the distances and angles between the transfer surfaces and so on will help the patient use the skill in novel circumstances. The second specific suggestion is that by interspersing a number of differing tasks randomly in one therapy session long-term retention will be facilitated — although at some cost to the immediate standard of performance. Therapists may wish to use blocked trials at first so that the patient gains an initial level of mastery and then progress to more variation (around a single task) and randomness (alternation between tasks) in the practice of skills.

COGNITIVE FACTORS

Over recent years evidence has been accruing for the significant role played by cognitive processes in the learning of motor behaviour. Cognitive factors have been shown to influence even apparently involuntary motor behaviour (Hammond, 1956; quoted in Stelmach and Diggles, 1982). The evidence for KR and KP, particularly when other forms of feedback are impaired, has already been discussed. Other factors such as rehearsal and labelling (Shea, 1977) may also be important in the subsequent recall of movement sequences. Cognitive rehearsal means repeating in imagination the performance of a movement either visually (in one's mind's eye) or verbally. Labelling means the naming of components of movements and then either the repetition of these labels out loud or using the labels sub-vocally. So, for example, learning a piece of classical ballet is made considerably easier by the fact that frequently used positions have names, e.g. an arabesque. Since the dancer already knows what physical movement is involved in an arabesque using these labels as verbal codes greatly facilitates the learning of a more complex piece, e.g. principal female in Swan Lake.

Having subjects describe their performance on a linear movement task has been demonstrated to aid recall (Ho and Shea, 1979) a result of which was explained with reference to Craik and Lockhart's (1972) depth of processing model. Other workers have found that set organisation of a task aids learning. Unfortunately almost all of the work examining these factors has been performed on children, or the non-neurologically impaired learning novel motor tasks, or on normals attempting to learn to control movements not usually under voluntary control (Balliet and Nakayama, 1978).

THERAPEUTIC IMPLICATIONS OF THEORIES OF MOTOR LEARNING

Open- and closed-loop models have differing implications for the control of already acquired motor patterns. Schmidt (1980), for example, has suggested that selection of feedback- or programme-based control depends on the task, the attentional requirements, the accuracy requirements and the level of training. However, for the therapist in the clinical setting, whether an overlearned movement is eventually controlled by closed- or open-loop mechanisms, acquisition of movements is likely to be closed-loop. Almost all activities can be taught more easily when the initial practice is slow and then with a gradual increase in speed rather than by attempting to train fast movements (Kottke, 1982; Bach-y-Rita et al., 1987). This will be particularly true as frequently increased effort can produce rapid degeneration in performance in patients with hypertonicity.

Despite the differences in theories of motor learning they all agree on the importance of practice, feedback, goal specificity, and motivational and attentional variables.

One of the most important factors in learning is practice. Our clinical experience suggests that, in the early stages, working in even a slightly different way will disrupt the learning process. However, once mastery has been achieved in the limited clinical environment the skill then needs to be practised in varied environments and in realistic situations. Therapists typically underestimate the amount of practice required to establish a stable response pattern. Because an individual can produce a response for half an hour a day in one setting when being supervised by a physical or occupational therapist does not mean that the individual can do the same thing all the time and in other settings. Practice reduces the effort necessary to initiate action. The patient not only needs to know how to perform but also must overlearn actual performance if the desired response is not to break down. Considerable overlearning needs to take place before a newly acquired skill can be produced automatically (first practise until you get it right then practise until you can't get it wrong). This suggests another important distinction: that between performance and learning. Therapists frequently use methods which improve the patient's performance immediately after their use, such as vibration or ice. These will, however, only have a limited effect unless either the techniques produce lasting (e.g. structural) results or the patient learns how to incorporate the method into day-to-day activities.

There are a number of indications that it may be useful to think of therapeutic interventions after brain injury as falling into two separate phases. The first is the acute recovery stage which frequently involves non-specific or stimulatory procedures designed to provoke the maximum in spontaneous recovery. The second category is the post-acute treatment which is reserved for cases where recovery has not achieved the level required for function and involves specific training. Both enhanced sensory feedback approaches and behavioural training programmes can be useful in this second category. Conductive education is probably unique in being able to function as a model for intervention in both phases of treatment.

CONDUCTIVE EDUCATION AS A MODEL OF PHYSICAL REHABILITATION

Current types of therapy frequently fail to teach the severely impaired brain-damaged adult improved motor performance. Due to the mode of presentation, patients with memory or attentional disorders cannot acquire the information they would need to improve their performance. This is for the very good reason that the patient's learning is of only incidental importance in many of these approaches. Unlike more standard approaches to physical rehabilitation, conductive education stresses the patient's active participation in treatment rather than the handling skill of the therapist (Cotton and Kinsman, 1983). Conductive education incorporates many of the factors which theories of motor learning suggest will enhance learning. For example because conductive education stresses the day's practical activities, not only can patients understand the importance of moving correctly, and using methods learned in daily tasks; they are also able to appreciate the results directly. Conductive education can serve as a model of physical rehabilitation for patients with severe brain injury.

Conductive education was developed by Professor Andras Peto, who founded the Institute for Conductive Education of the Motor Disabled and Conductors College in Budapest in 1945 (Cotton, 1965; Holt, 1975). It is an educational approach to the treatment of physical disabilities arising from neurological impairment.

The use of a group is central to the approach. The groups differ in function — but the aims of the group are to practise motor tasks and improve the patient's performance on them. A task series, composed of the separate elements of the task, are written by the conductor according to the needs of the patient. The conductor states the movement, the patients repeat it and perform the appropriate action whilst counting. In this way a complex task is built up from small movements. A second conductor moves around the group directing attention to areas of difficulty and providing assistance if required. The session ends with all the patients performing the task. Thus the first conductor writes and presents the programme and delivers instructions, feedback and praise. The second conductor must know the programme, the patients, and the amount of facilitation the patient requires. The conductor's task is to stimulate the

Table 7.1: Aim: To pick objects up from the floor

1. I sit ready	
Introductions – Good mornings, etc. Explain purpose of class	
2. Two flat feet	1,2,3,4,5
3. Clasp hands together	1,2,3,4,5
4. Stretch elbows	1,2,3,4,5
5. Look at straight elbows	1,2,3,4,5
6. Hands inside out	1,2,3,4,5
7. Hands to floor	1,2,3,4,5
8. Thumbs together	1,2,3,4,5
9. Separate hands	1,2,3,4,5
(put object, e.g. paper towel, next to hands)	
10. Pick up towel	1,2,3,4,5
11. Sit up	1,2,3,4,5
12. I sit ready	1,2,3,4,5
Now try the same thing with one hand.	
13. Left hand to left foot	1,2,3,4,5
14. Sit up	1,2,3,4,5
15. Left hand to right foot	1,2,3,4,5
16. Sit up	1,2,3,4,5
17. Left hand between feet	1,2,3,4,5
18. Sit up	1,2,3,4,5
19. Right hand to right foot	1,2,3,4,5
20. Sit up	1,2,3,4,5
21. Right hand to left foot	1,2,3,4,5
22. Sit up	1,2,3,4,5
23. Right hand between feet	1,2,3,4,5
24. Sit up	1,2,3,4,5
Discuss which is the easiest method, etc.	

patient to achieve the maximum amount of independence in all settings (Holt, 1975).

FACILITATIONS TO LEARNING

There are a number of key elements in conductive education.

(1) All therapy is aimed towards a functional goal. Assessment is in terms of the patient's ability to carry out basic functional tasks: (a) rolling, (b) sitting, (c) standing, (d) walking, (e) feeding, (f) washing, (g) dressing, (h) toileting, and (i) writing (or equivalent fine motor task). Similarly patients are taught methods to sit, stand, eat, walk or write.

(2) Each functional task is broken down into component steps that are discrete, understandable, and achievable (with or without facilitation). In this way the approach is made both goal-directed and achievement-oriented.

(3) Each functional task is carried out with the aid of verbal regulation: the individual states his intention to perform a task and then performs the task whilst monitoring his performance verbally.

(4) Conductive education is a total treatment approach in that skills initially established in sessions are then practised in a vast number of other situations so that eventually the skill becomes automatic.

(5) Conductive education is an interdisciplinary team approach and requires the involvement of all members of the team.

Since conductive education is conceptualised as a learning approach the various techniques used are thought of as facilitations to learning.

TASK ANALYSIS

In conductive education functional tasks are broken down into finite achievable steps which are then carried out using whatever facilitations are required to achieve a normal motor pattern. Movement starts with an intention and ends with a goal. The intention to carry out the task is invariant. The solution to the achievement of the task may be varied. The goal is invariant. For example the intention to drink from a cup is always the same; there are many different ways to hold a cup and to transport it to the mouth, but if successful the result is always the same, getting the cup to the mouth. When working towards the development of any individual function it is first necessary to carry out a task analysis of the normal pattern of movement.

To teach the task it is necessary to:

(a) conceptualise the task — by demonstration or verbal explanation;
(b) build the movements into subgoals;
(c) build the subgoals into the goal.

Table 7.2: Example of a task analysis

(a) Identify the goal
(b) Break the goal down into subgoals
(c) Break the subgoals down into movements

Drinking from a cup

Subgoals could be: To sit well; to grasp cup; to take cup to mouth

Subgoal 'To sit well':
1. Feet flat
2. Bottom back
3. Back straight
4. Head in the mid-line
5. Hands flat on the table

Subgoal 'To grasp cup':
1. To make a fist
2. To bring out thumb
3. To bring out index finger
4. To bring out middle finger
5. To make a tripod grasp
6. To pick up cup

Subgoal 'To take cup to mouth'
1. To keep flat hand still
2. To look at cup
3. To take cup to mouth
4. To drink from cup

INDIVIDUAL FACILITATIONS

In order to carry out a particular task the patient may need facilitation, either by incorporating the use of equipment into the task, or from the conductor.

The conductor controls enough of the variables and provides enough facilitation to guarantee some measure of success. However, the completion of the task should incorporate the patient's maximum effort at that stage in treatment. In this way the patient can learn what is correct about his or her performance.

1. Self-facilitation

(a) Gravity: the patient learns to inhibit spasticity by letting his hands hang down, thereby increasing the chances of easier performance of the task.

(b) Self-positioning: the patient learns to position himself so as to inhibit mass patterns of movement and/or spasticity.

(c) Self-handling: the patient may need to inhibit spasticity by, for example, clasping hands together whilst protracting the scapulae and straightening the elbows.

In conjunction with the conductor, the patient can develop and incorporate his own methods of inhibiting spasticity into the task. A piece of furniture or equipment can be useful in the inhibition of spasticity, gaining symmetry, or performing a movement.

2. Conductor facilitation

The patient may only need to have his attention directed towards a movement or aspect of positioning in order to accomplish a task. In this case the conductor simply points or, if necessary, touches the patient as a prompt. The most difficult task for the patient may be the inhibition of unwanted movement, which may depend to a large degree on the allocation of attentional resources. In some cases the conductor may need to provide fixation of a body part for the patient to be able to carry out the required movement. For example for the patient to abduct the right leg in lying, it may be necessary for the conductor to help hold the left leg still. At other times the patient may require physical facilitation in performing a movement. The facilitation provided should be the minimum to allow the successful completion of the task.

Verbal feedback is frequently provided during the session. It is highly specific in form and efforts are made to ensure that it is always encouraging. The conductor says a performance was good and then why. 'Great, Paul! You had a good hip bend in transferring,' or 'Good, David, you kept your head up when you took that step.' If a patient is performing a task well, time out from the group task can be taken to allow the patient to demonstrate their performance to other group members. Patients are also frequently encouraged to make use of visual feedback. Sometimes this visual feedback is incorporated in the programme itself, e.g. 'I look at my straight elbows.'

THE USE OF THE GROUP

The use of the group is central to conductive education. Peer support and peer pressure are strong motivators. The conductor should find methods to enhance the effects of these factors.

LANGUAGE AND LEARNING

As discussed in an earlier part of this chapter, language can act to facilitate learning in a number of ways. An individual frequently instructs himself in words, thereby increasing his ability to complete a task or to learn a skill. As the skill is learned the verbal regulation is gradually internalised (Fitts and Posner, 1967). This can be seen in adults particularly when trying to acquire a complex task such as learning how to play a musical instrument or drive a car. Although the evidence as to the importance of speech in this process is unclear, language is clearly implicated in the learning and retention of motor output (Adams, 1971, 1976). Verbal regulation is a key element in conductive education. This procedure incorporates two elements: (1) rhythmical intention and (2) speech regulation. Together, these elements may aid motor organisation and planning, and may act to inhibit unwanted motor activity (Luria, 1961). For example, the first conductor gives the instruction, e.g. 'I make two flat hands.' The patient and instructor together then repeat the instruction 'I make two flat hands', and the movement is then performed to a count (one, two). The rhythm can be varied to the needs of the patient. Some additional advantages to the use of language in this patient population include:

(1) increased arousal,
(2) increased attention to task,
(3) reduced effect of external auditory distractions.

During the sessions the conductor needs to be dynamic and to impose a vigorous rhythm, both to hold the patient's attention and to maintain the patient's level of arousal (a slow 1–5 count is used when inhibiting spasticity or when carrying out a difficult task). The phrases used in the rhythmical intention must be ·

short to aid ease of repetition and to ensure a high level of comprehension. To a limited degree one could regard the verbal regulation as a narration which can enhance learning by directing the patients' attention to the significant aspects of their performance. If patients do not selectively attend to the critical aspects of the programme they will find it more difficult to reproduce the behaviour.

The conductor needs to know how much speech to expect from a dysarthric patient. Over-expectation will mean that the patient will have to direct too much attention to his speech, at the expense of movement. The patient with receptive dysphasia may need to have movements modelled for him by the conductor or by other group participants, or to have the verbal regulation tailored to his needs. As with dysarthric patients, the patient with dysphasia should only be expected to use verbal regulation if it does not interfere with being able to perform the physical movement.

CONCLUSION

Two separate elements coexist in physical rehabilitation after brain injury. These elements overlap but at their extremes are quite distinct. Here we will call these elements strategies and motor output. Strategies refer to how patients organise their behaviour in order to overcome the functional handicaps arising from physical deficits. So, for example, patients might learn how to inhibit unwanted motor responses, organise a transfer, or position themselves so as to have a stable sitting position. Motor output, on the other hand, involves the ease, fluency and control of movement. Rehabilitation approaches stress either one element or the other. Many therapists dislike adopting the first approach for fear of not stimulating the patient to the best possible physical recovery. Opting for the second approach, however, runs the risk of leaving the patient after intensive therapy without necessary functional skills. Conductive education can help therapists overcome these conflicts by combining both approaches. Conductive education encourages patients to adopt functional problem-solving strategies which maximise stimulation and foster improved motor output.

8

Education for the Severely Impaired Brain-injured Adult

Jill Edney

Knowledge basic to functioning in society is frequently absent in the severely brain-injured adult. In some cases this seems to be as a direct result of the brain injury. In other cases knowledge is deficient as an indirect result of the injury, such as when schooling was interrupted by trauma and the individual was lost to the educational system. Many patients may have had poor academic histories prior to injury. In many cases cognitive deficits such as dysphasia or memory impairments hamper performance, and the individual must learn new strategies in order to perform tasks which were previously accomplished easily. Unfortunately cognitive deficits mean that it is often very difficult for the brain-injured patient to acquire new skills, so that the teacher must devote considerable ingenuity to deciding not only what to teach, but how to present information so that the individual can make use of it. Areas of cognitive deficit may include attention and concentration, impulsiveness, memory impairment, concrete thinking, difficulty in initiating behaviour, impaired problem-solving, disinhibition and perseveration.

Unlike work with the paediatric population, where the aim is frequently to reintegrate the patient into the educational system, the teacher's role with adults is to help them become as independent as possible. This may or may not include returning to work, depending upon the patient's degree of impairment.

If the patient received the injury as an adult, an educational and vocational history may help establish the limits of likely improvement.

The teacher can offer assessment and teaching of the basic skills of reading, writing and arithmetic, and the use of these skills in a practical setting. The teacher also offers knowledge about day-to-day life skills (such as how to use a post office). Often in conjunction with therapists in other disciplines the teacher can help patients develop social and recreational skills.

ASSESSMENT

Most programmes described in the literature (Cohen *et al.*, 1985; Cohen, S.B., 1986) describe work with adolescents, whereas this chapter focuses on the adult post-acute population. During an initial assessment period the patient's behaviour, motivation and abilities are observed. The patient may also have been included in some individual and group sessions and asked to participate, thus informal assessment is continuously taking place. As problems become evident team members will communicate these to each other, with appropriate advice on how best to handle them. The speech therapist will advise on a patient with severe communication problems, and the teacher will advise on reading and writing ability. Communication between team members is essential to achieve an integrated picture of the patient.

There is no educational assessment which is applicable to the whole range of problems encountered in working with the brain-injured adult. A series of simple assignments can be used to gauge the performance of patients in basic skills. For the purposes of assessment, reading and arithmetic skills need to be broken down into their component parts so that if a patient has difficulty with a particular area it can be probed further. It also highlights the areas of deficiency in which the patient would benefit from further instruction. The patient's performance must be recorded so that subsequent comparisons can be made. Of necessity assessment is sometimes by informal testing. Changes in performance must be assessed, but the process of assessment should not be so frequent or time-consuming that it hampers treatment.

Assessment of basic skills aims to define abilities in reading, writing, comprehension, basic arithmetic and the ability to handle money and tell time. Comprehension of written language is closely related to comprehension of verbal language. Where initial assessment indicates a deficit a sample of an individual's writing prior to injury is useful. Often injury may make a pre-existing dyslexia more pronounced. Where the reading disorder appears to be acquired as a result of injury the teacher should consult a speech therapist to determine if the deficit is unique to reading, or if it parallels a language disorder. A discussion of the various types of alexias is beyond the scope of this chapter and the interested reader is referred to the work of Friedman and Alpert (1985). When examining reading, a note should be taken of whether the individual 'sounds out' each word, indicating an inability to read words as complete units (surface alexia), or whether the individual is unable to sound out words (phonological alexia), as this may affect the type of intervention employed. The ability to read should not be mistaken for the ability to comprehend printed material, nor should the inability to read aloud be mistaken for the inability to comprehend printed material. Problems with writing (agraphia) are also a frequent phenomenon but not necessarily concomitant with alexia.

Major deficits in mathematical skills are most frequently due to either absence of premorbid ability or cognitive deficits which affect arithmetic ability, such as disturbances of memory and attention. For a discussion of specific acalculic syndromes the reader is referred to Levin and Spiers (1985).

Reading and writing assessment 'tool kit'

When conducting an assessment it is helpful to have on hand a selection of material that can be employed as the need arises. A useful 'tool kit' for assessment of reading and writing skills includes a short passage of five or six sentences of moderate reading difficulty presented in normal-sized print and the same passage in larger print for patients with sight difficulties. In addition a range of short passages of written material of increasing complexity can be used to assess the abilities of higher-functioning patients. Also in the 'tool kit' should be pictures and words to match; upper and lower case alphabet cards; pictures and sentences to match; a set of functional signs (e.g. toilet, exit, open, men); a set of shapes; a telephone directory; a form requiring personal information and a selection of writing materials. For the severely handicapped patient, thick felt-tipped pens and large paper may be needed.

In the initial assessment the patient is asked to read the passage aloud, and then again to himself so he is able to answer questions. He will then write the passage to dictation. If previous observation has shown the patient incapable of functioning at this level, the assessment will begin at a place judged to be more appropriate. Reading and writing to dictation exercise will show any deficiencies in reading ability, comprehension, spelling and writing which will be recorded and explored further. If a patient completes these exercises successfully he will then be asked to apply these skills to more functional tasks, such as finding a given name and address in the telephone directory and filling in a simple form. Subsequent sessions and assessments will put the patient in more demanding situations until his level of ability is ascertained.

If the patient is having difficulties reading the passage or, after initial attempts, refuses to cooperate, it will be necessary to break the task down into small sections and carefully record achievements and areas of difficulty. For the more seriously impaired patient it is necessary to begin with the most simple tasks and build up to the more complex. It is essential to give the patient an opportunity to succeed, and thus build his confidence and self-esteem and gain his cooperation. Other uses for the reading and writing 'tool kit' are shown in Table 8.1.

Table 8.1: Ancillary uses for the 'tool kit'

Identifying pictures of named objects
Matching picture with written word
Putting the alphabet in the correct order
Recognising and naming letters
Cross-case matching
Indicating the initial letter/sound of a word
Following simple written instructions, e.g. Point to the card
   with the flower on it and pick up the pencil
Spelling high-frequency words (oral and written)
Matching sentences and pictures
Reading different parts of speech (e.g. concrete nouns,
   abstract nouns, verbs, adjectives, and function words)
Recognition of functional signs
Free writing (such as describing a picture)
Copying letters, words and sentences
Writing name and address and signature

A vast range of problems are found in the area of reading and spelling in the head-injured population, and are shown in Table 8.2.

Table 8.2: Reading and spelling problems experienced by head-injured patients

The ability to recognise familiar words such as names of relatives and meaningful nouns (e.g. milk, tea, coffee) but an inability to express them
Inability to read function words (e.g. in, the, and, was, there)
Inability to use phonetics
Inability to recognise a whole word unless it can be built up phonetically
Inability to read due to premorbid lack of education
Changing letter-order of words, or substituting similar-sounding word when reading, e.g. 'stop' is read as 'spot'
The word-order of the sentence is changed, thus rendering it nonsense
Ability to read but inability to spell
Missing out words on one side of the paper due to visual inattention or hemianopia
Ability to read large print, but unable to make use of it for functional or pleasure purposes due to visual difficulties (consultation with a neuro-ophthalmologist required)
Ability to read but inability to comprehend what is read

Mathematics assessment 'tool kit'

The 'tool kit' for basic mathematics, money and time consists of: cubes, counters, or other items to count; number recognition cards; simple arithmetic equations in the four rules to be presented in both oral and written forms (e.g. $5 + 2 =$), a selection of coins and currency, a clock, a watch, a timetable and a calendar.

Patients who prove themselves to be competent in simple tasks can be assessed on their ability to complete more complex mathematical exercises.

Liquid, weight and line measurement are of secondary importance in functional living compared to money and time, and therefore do not need to be included in an initial assessment. Patients who demonstrate that their basic mathematical concepts are intact will have the opportunity to improve these skills when involved in functional activities such as budgeting, cooking, and reading maps and timetables.

During assessment the patient's manner and cooperation, and any behaviour which prevents him from achieving the completion of tasks, is noted and recorded. His level of communication will also be ascertained, from social greetings to the ability to converse and express an opinion. Assessment

153

Table 8.3: More advanced exercises

Recognition and naming of written numbers: (a) 1–10, (b) 11–20, (c) over 20

Counting a number of dots and objects

Automatic counting 1–100

Matching number of objects with numbers

Understanding ordinal numbers — 1st, 2nd, etc.

Understand and correct use of such concepts as more than/less than, smallest/largest

Simple arithmetic equations, addition, subtraction, multiplication and division; presented in oral and written form

Recognition and naming of coins and currency

Knowledge of relative value of coins

Addition of given amounts of money

Appropriate handling of money in a shopping situation

Solving of simple money problems (make change)

Use of a calendar and understanding of terms such as yesterday, tomorrow, last week

Use of a 12-hour clock face

Use of a digital clock and can count 12 hour to 24 hour

Use of a timetable

---

results and observations are discussed by the team members. Problem areas are defined and prioritised according to the needs of the patient. A treatment programme can then be initiated using behavioural methods similar to those outlined in other chapters of this book.

HANDWRITING

Patients may have impaired writing skills due to physical and visual difficulties, inability to inhibit actions (perseveration) and the inability to initiate actions as well as alexia. Consultation with the physiotherapist or occupational therapist is necessary to ensure correct sitting position and grasp of writing implement in order to gain maximum control, and therefore achieve the best results. Patients with visuospatial deficits have difficulty judging distance from pen to paper. Their writing is usually faint and spidery. Practice is required to achieve the correct pen pressure on the paper to form legible handwriting.

The following activities are useful exercises for practising motor control: joining a line of dots, tracing over letters, copying underneath letters.

Production of upper-case letters is easier than lower-case as the lines and curves required are more manageable. When the upper- and lower-case letters have been mastered, cursive writing can be tackled. The order of difficulty of upper-case letters is: letters using only horizontal and vertical lines (E, F, H, L, T, I); those including diagonal lines (A, K, M, N, V, W, X, Z, Y); anticlockwise movement (C, G, O, Q, S, U); and clockwise movement (B, D, J, P, R). Lower-case letters can be split into similar groupings.

The aim of treatment is to produce functional handwriting. If a patient is able to print legibly he should be encouraged to use it functionally while practising cursive writing in a more formal manner. Some 'fun and functional' handwriting activities are:

(1) Making boxes. A game to be played in a group. Each person joins two dots. The person who joins the final two dots to complete a box claims it by putting his initials in the box. The winner is whoever initials the most boxes.
(2) Noughts and crosses.
(3) Crossword puzzles.
(4) Writing signature on Christmas and birthday cards.
(5) Writing shopping lists.
(6) Filling in forms.
(7) Writing letters and addressing envelopes.
(8) Drawing and sketching.

A number of patients have been seen who are unable to inhibit movements (perseveration) and require a behavioural learning programme to enable them to control their writing. Their writing may get smaller and smaller until it deteriorates into one long line, or one letter may be repeated many times with many unnecessary dots and meaningless 'squiggles'. A special programme incorporating clear directions for when to stop (e.g. after each word, after each letter) may help patients produce more functional writing.

For the most severely handicapped patients the aim will be to write or sign their name legibly and consistently to be accepted by a bank. For patients who are well preserved cognitively but who, due to severe physical disabilities, cannot write by hand, other methods for obtaining written communication may need to be explored. A typewriter, microwriter, or a computer word processing programme with adapted controls may be suitable for such patients.

READING AND SPELLING

After the teacher has ascertained the patient's baseline abilities, and the areas and degree of the problem, an appropriate programme of instruction can be instituted. Patients who are able to use phonetics benefit from a word-building programme involving:

(1) Teaching letter names and sounds.
(2) Identifying initial sounds of words (simple games can be made up to make learning fun).
(3) Learning consonant blends (for example: th, ch, sh, st) and identifying these blends in words (for example: with, church, this).
(4) Vowel sounds a, e, i. o, u. Words can be built using the sounds learned (for example: shop, stop, cat, bat, sat).
(5) Vowel sounds, orthographically represented by double letters (oo, ee, ea) can be built using these combinations (for example: moon, sheep, sea, tea).
(6) The addition of 'r' changes the vowel sound; for example: ir, ur, er.
(7) Addition of 'magic "e" ' changes the vowel — mat becomes mate.
(8) Learning word endings (for example: -tion, -ing, -ed).

As many words do not adhere strictly to word-building rules, and therefore cannot be systematically built up, a different method must be used to learn them. The whole word must be presented and practised until it is learned.

It is important to break the process down to a level where the patient can achieve success as this maintains and increases motivation.

Patients who cannot use phonetics, because of their brain damage, may be able to learn to read using the sightword method. Words may be presented individually or in groups.

Using this method the patient is shown the whole word on a flash card (one word to each card) and repeats it after the instructor. Only two or three words should be instructed initially. Words which are particularly relevant to the patient will have the best chance of being retained. As the patient earns new words more can be added. In the group method, four or five words to be learned are printed in a line across the page. The same words are printed for five lines in a different order each time.

and	in	the	I
in	and	I	the
I	the	in	I
the	I	and	in
and	in	the	I

The instructor points to and says each word, and the student repeats it. At the appropriate time roles are reversed and the student reads the words first. This process continues until the student is able to read the words confidently. Other reading exercises and games can be used to practise words learned.

Simple sentences can be written out with each word on a separate card. The patient has to sort the sentence into the correct order. As mentioned previously, a topic relevant to the patient is preferable.

Completing a sentence with an appropriate word

    I drink ———
    My name is ———

Matching words to pictures and objects.

For those able to use phonetics making words is appropriate. Cut up words into parts for word-building sh/op, sh/eep, b/oy.

Sorting out simple sentences into correct order, e.g.

    I got out of bed.
    I got dressed.
    I went outside.

Reading-books can be made up by the patient about himself or anything he is interested in. It may only be a word and picture to begin with. Words learned can then be used in sentences.

For the patient with severe expressive language difficulties simple reading tasks enable the teacher to assess reading ability, e.g. matching the word 'milk' to a carton of milk, sorting jumbled words into sentences and matching names to people. The teacher should have either objects, or photographs of a range of objects, available. Where the patient is a non-speaker the teacher can work with the speech therapist in selecting and training the patient in the use of a communication aid, the complexity of which will depend on the patient's abilities.

Learning to read was a very stimulating activity for M.R., a 24-year-old young man who sustained a head injury when six years old and was handicapped by physical, visual and behavioural problems. M.R. had received some special schooling, but due to aggressive, antisocial behaviour he learned very little. M.R. knew some letter names and sounds and could read three words, 'is', 'and' and 'I'. As he was very keen to learn to read it was felt some instruction would be beneficial. After a year he was able to build up regular words using phonetics, and had a sight vocabulary of approximately 30 words. Practice in word-building was done with words he might find useful when in the community.

GROUP WORK

Working in groups can provide a greater level of stimulation than individual work, and allows the teacher to reinforce appropriate cooperation and behaviour with greater effect. The group can create a cohesive, secure atmosphere which is conducive to learning. To achieve this atmosphere groups must remain stable for a considerable period of time. With severely handicapped patients we have found between three and five patients a good number. Those with a severe language handicap will need the simple word–object, word–picture matching exercises already discussed. Counting objects and recognising numbers, identifying letters of the alphabet and identifying coins are all valuable areas to be worked on. A useful visual aid is a large calendar with removable pieces. Such concepts as day, month, year, yesterday, tomorrow can be practised. It is also valuable for counting and number recognition.

Improving listening, reading, comprehension and mathematical skills is necessary for those with impaired information processing. Group sessions are very effective in producing a competitive atmosphere which raises the level of arousal, and consequently the level of performance. Quick mental arithmetic and quizzes demanding short answers are very effective in producing an atmosphere of competition.

These group sessions are valuable occasions for the speech therapist and teacher to work together, particularly with those who have gross speech and language problems. Besides ensuring consistency and continuity both therapists can work on their particular areas within the group framework.

For patients with a higher level of language functioning videos, newspapers and magazines can be used to provoke discussions and maintain an interest in current affairs. Play-reading addresses a number of high-order skills, reading and listening, but also voice inflection, and helps develop understanding of social interaction. Choice of material is important. Topical and humorous material is more popular than the classics.

FUNCTIONAL APPLICATIONS OF EDUCATIONAL SKILLS

The patient who is able to read and write must learn to apply

Table 8.4: Areas needing training and practice

Appropriate use of telephone directory and telephone
Reading, comprehending and completing forms
Letter-writing, including appropriate greetings and conclusions for business or friendly letters; addressing envelopes correctly
Making lists (e.g. a shopping list)
Reading, comprehending and applying instructions, e.g. a recipe book or directions on a food packet
Using a bus or train timetable and use of TV/radio guides
Understanding money, budgeting, how to use a bank account, writing cheques
Supermarket pricing and labelling; ways of using a supermarket as opposed to smaller shops; finding food items on shelves
Clothes sizing and labelling
Weighing items for cooking

these skills in functional situations. Cooperation between teacher and occupational therapist is necessary to ascertain areas needing specific instruction, and to ensure that the particular needs of each patient are being met. Training and practice are often needed, in those areas shown in Table 8.4, to help the patient towards functional independence.

J.B.R., a 29-year-old male engineering graduate, wished to increase his functional independence but was hampered by acquired dyslexia, a severe memory problem, and a specific agnosia for fruit and vegetables. J.B.R. had retained good reasoning abilities, which were harnessed to help him overcome his memory problems. The occupational therapist was training J.B.R. to cook for himself, but found reading and understanding instructions, including such terms as boil and grill, were proving difficult. Extra practice in understanding these terms and reading lists of instructions was needed without actually having to cook.

Handling money is a skill necessary for independent living. Even if help and advice are at hand some knowledge of, and ability to handle, your own money gives a boost to confidence and self-esteem. Patients who are able to recognise the name and value of coins can be encouraged to give an appropriate amount of money in a given situation, e.g. when buying a 30p chocolate bar a 50p coin is more appropriate than a 5 pound note. It is important to use 'real' money rather than imitation money as the weight, feel and shape of real money needs to be continuously experienced if patients are to feel confident about using it. Many patients are not familiar with the one pound coin; the 20p and 5p pieces in particular give many problems in identification. Finding and reading price labels in shops and supermarkets provides good practice for reading numbers, scanning along shelves, identifying food items, and appreciating the value of money. A small selection of items can be used for practice sessions before the actual shopping excursion. Terms such as 'cheapest' and 'most expensive' can be taught, and practice provided in mental and written arithmetic, depending on the abilities of the group. Such questions as 'How much more expensive is the coffee than the tea bags?' or 'How much change will I have from 5 pounds if I spend 3 pounds 50p?' provide practice in reasoning, comprehension and arithmetic and language skills. On returning from a shopping trip money and shopping bills can be checked to ascertain if the correct change was given. It is also a good opportunity to weigh fruit and vegetable items and identify weight on the shop labels. A good relationship with the local shops is invaluable.

Books such as *Maths in print*, *Maths about town*, and *Maths about the shops* by Bill Ridgeway, published by Edward Arnold, have practical exercises in the functional use of maths for more able patients. Unfortunately the print is rather small for those with visual deficits, but they provide some good ideas which could be used for work sheets. They also produce an informative package containing ideas for work sheets, called *Using the Post Office*. Simple arithmetic work books provide good practice and can be used either for oral or written work. Patients gain satisfaction from having their work corrected and improving on their scores.

In higher-functioning patients where money management may present problems an account book recording income and expenditure can be kept. The book should be balanced at the end of every week. If the patient is going to be using a bank and cheque book time should be given to research, compare and learn how banks operate and the advantages of using them. Literature from various banking institutions can be collected and discussed, and patients can become familiar with such terms used to describe the types of accounts. Using a cheque book and banker's card needs to be explained and practised. If appropriate, it is a valuable exercise for the patient to open an account with the bank of his/her choice and learn how to use it under supervision. It may be necessary to approach the family and/or social worker and explain the advantages of the patient handling his own money to make this possible. This exercise was successfully achieved with a patient who preferred to hide her money in her room. It is a necessary learning experience for a person working towards taking control of his or her own life.

When letter-writing, using a telephone and telephone directory, and reading maps and timetables have been mastered as individual activities, they then need to be practised in a functional setting. They are the lines of communications and enquiry which enable us to achieve a further objective. Such a programme was embarked upon by P.G. and S.B., both of whom were able to function at a high level but needed guidance to integrate into the community. P.G. in particular had spent several years, from her mid-teens, in a hospital, and lacked confidence when faced with the prospect of independent living.

They both had no idea of how to research the facilities outside the sphere of the hospital. After discussion a plan of action was drawn up and worked through.

A trip to the local library and advice bureau revealed names and addresses of clubs and organisations. Each then had to formulate a list of the information they needed and decide which method of enquiry they were going to employ. In practice both letter-writing and telephoning were used. The resulting information then had to be evaluated as to the suitability for their individual needs. This entailed consulting local maps and bus timetables, asking themselves such questions as:

Can I reach the club by bus?
How long will it take me?
Can I afford to go by taxi?
Is the meeting at a time I can go regularly?

Both P.G. and S.B. achieved their aim, and found suitable clubs catering for their particular interests: drama and French conversation. Support and encouragement was still needed as lack of confidence when meeting others was the biggest hurdle to overcome. S.B. is now living in her own house with a companion, and P.G. is hoping to do the same in the near future. The teacher must be aware of the capabilities and the needs of the patient, and must give the patient the best opportunity to put his abilities to functional use.

LEISURE

The severely brain-injured adult who is unlikely to resume a full-time job will need activities and interests to occupy his time. The lack of motivation to initiate activities is a problem which has to be overcome, so participating in leisure activities is an important part of rehabilitation. Patients initially need to be introduced to several activities and asked to participate. Eventually they may be motivated to initiate an activity without prompting from others.

GAMES

For people whose lives are limited by any disability, board

games provide valuable opportunities for social interaction. Playing games with one other person or in a group gives an opportunity to apply language, mathematical, reasoning and social skills. Besides practising skills, patients are able to experience and become confident in activities which are acceptable in all sections of society.

Table 8.5: Skills required to play scrabble or dominoes

Eye/hand coordination	Physical control	Reading and spelling
To place pieces in correct place	Manipulating pieces	To make words
Scanning while observing play	Attention and concentration	Reasoning and information processing Following instructions
	Passing pieces (incorporating social skills in turn-taking)	

MUSIC AND BOOKS

Many people enjoy music, books or magazines of some description. For those with severe sight deficits, and who have lost the ability to read, listening can become a valued activity. The public library is a source of tapes of comedy shows, music of all varieties and talking books. Patients who were avid readers prior to their accident, but have since lost the ability or motivation to read, often regain their interest through talking books. A library visit to select books and tapes, combined with a stop at a nearby restaurant, can make a purposeful visit out.

Large-print books are also available. These books are adult in content but some have large, bright, glossy pictures and can stimulate interest in non-readers and provide good subjects for discussion. The pictures are fun to look at and talk about. It is important for the patient to feel involved in choosing his own listening and reading matter, and perhaps to build up a rapport with the local library as a pleasant place to visit.

Reading for pleasure was a hobby C.G. enjoyed prior to his accident. C.G. was physically and verbally aggressive, and visual difficulties prevented him from attempting to read anything. Large-print novels and a newsprint magnifying glass

163

were given to C.G., who was uncooperative, claiming he couldn't see. After several attempts to interest him he read half a page aloud. C.G. was socially reinforced for his achievement. He was asked to read half a page aloud every day, and was given social praise if he achieved the task. Gradually the length of the amount to be read was extended until C.G. was reading for an hour to himself. He found he was beginning to enjoy his books and began to take books to read in his own time.

COMPUTER

A computer can be used by even the severely physically impaired with special adaptations such as concept keyboards, joy sticks and switches. The many games, ranging over a wide ability level, provide another avenue to be explored when considering hobbies. A number of excellent programs are available for developing simple mathematics and reading skills.

GARDENING

Gardening can become a rewarding hobby, giving an opportunity for a handicapped person to participate in a 'normal' activity and providing a vehicle for practice of physical and cognitive skills. A gardening group can stimulate communication and social interaction. Sitting round a table planting seeds, or potting plants, demands cooperation and communication. There is also the satisfaction of seeing plants grow and producing flowers, fruit and vegetables. Such activities as flower arranging, making cress sandwiches or lettuce soup can follow on when the gardening begins to produce results.

Patients who show particular interest may like to have responsibility for their own small cactus garden or bottle garden. Those who are able to do more than window-sill gardening may enjoy cultivating a small plot outside. Large tubs provide accessible areas to cultivate. A flower competition stimulates extra interest and motivation.

ARTS AND CRAFTS

Painting, drawing, leatherwork, clay modelling and many other crafts can be practised as individual or group projects. As with gardening, a joint project can stimulate conversation and an awareness of other people, as well as providing ample opportunity to practise physical and cognitive skills. Patients also enjoy the feeling of satisfaction when an item has been completed and can be admired. For those who show particular interest and aptitude it can become an absorbing hobby.

The following are useful books for practising language skills:

Headword Book 1–4 (Oxford University Press).
What the papers said, by Redvers Brandling (Edward Arnold).
Would you believe it? by Redvers Brandling (Edward Arnold).
Stories and Plays. Spirals (Hutchinson).
Writing retraining: a systematic workbook, by C. Mazzella-Gordon and Z.A. Siepser (in press).

9

The Social and Emotional Consequences of Severe Brain Injury: The Social Work Perspective

Mary Lees

INTRODUCTION

Severe brain injury will always have serious implications for the person and his or her relatives, and in some cases cause drastic changes to many people's lives.

For many a sudden event, often a road traffic accident, changes lives considerably. The very nature of brain damage means that the person's intellectual, emotional and physical functioning will be impaired, often seriously. Inevitably, both for the brain-injured person and all who are involved, relationships will alter and adjustments have to be made. This chapter will consider reactions of brain-injured patients and their relatives to the consequences of the injury, and will describe and comment on individual solutions. Illustrations will be provided where both social work and clinical team involvement may be of help to patient and family.

NEEDS OF THE FAMILY IN THE ACUTE STAGE

Brain injury results in a sudden change in the life of both the injured individual and his or her family. The usual circumstances involve an emergency, or crisis affecting family and friends. They have to make immediate changes in routine daily life to allow for long periods of time to be spent at a hospital. Initially there are many offers of practical assistance for most families. The whole focus is on recovery: parents, spouses and children sit by the bed of a person who is in a coma, trying to rouse him or her by, for example, talking about familiar people and events and playing music. Family or friends, though shocked and upset, have clear roles. It is unlikely at this stage that future care is discussed, and relatives comment that they either received no information or advice, or that which they did receive was unacceptable. Distressed relatives, told that someone may never walk or talk again, are often determined to fight, not believing such a prognosis about a loved one. This reaction can lead to emotional difficulties in the later rehabilitative stage, as discussed later in this chapter, when relatives who have been deeply involved find it difficult to relinquish the role which has become a necessary way of life. In particular if a patient does make recovery in some areas despite an initially cautious prognosis, relatives, feeling medical staff were wrong, continue to work towards total recovery, unable to accept inevitable limitations and problems.

It may not be possible to provide helpful and specific information, because of the difficulty surgeons may have in predicting the outcome, and because of their unwillingness to do so when individuals are so vulnerable. The family may be unable to accept such information, denying reality. It would be helpful at this time to convey hopeful but realistic facts to the family. Information about outcome, related to specific areas of brain injury, is becoming more available and needs to be documented and accessible to all clinical staff involved in intensive care and surgical units, to general practitioners and to patients' families. By illustrating the wide range of possible degrees of recovery, the number of years likely to be involved and other factors it should be possible to give families cautiously hopeful but realistic information. Family relationships and interactions are a vital issue in rehabilitation, and it would be helpful to persuade relatives at an early stage that there are several possibilities implicit in recovery. Nothing is gained by giving too little or too much hope at the time of injury, and such pronouncements are often remembered and are the source of later bitterness, damaging to the relationship between patient, family and treatment teams.

It is essential that the family receive immediate counselling, support and assistance, and that a hospital social worker becomes involved with all brain-injured patients and their families as soon as is practicable. In some intensive-care or treatment units social workers are called in for immediate contact, and this should be standard practice. The family should be able to meet and talk with members of the treatment team, but it is the social worker who most easily adopts the role of counsellor. There are practical arrangements to be made, and legal and financial advice should be given even at an early stage. It is surprising how often families remain unaware of the social security benefits to which the patient is entitled, so efforts should be made to ensure that groundwork towards the eventual securing of such benefits goes on, even when the family may have immense difficulty in looking ahead. Families must also be advised to care for the health of all the members involved at this stressful period.

If the patient makes reasonable physical progress he or she is often discharged home. Social work involvement must continue in the community. It is not unusual that families are discovered, living with the difficulties produced by the brain-injured person, with little support and with problems compounding an already stressful situation (Livingston, 1986b). It is not surprising that social workers may lack the specialist information needed, and the brain-injured person may not appear to require the services of psychiatric or mental handicap teams as readily as those of the physical handicap teams. Yet it is when the brain-injured person goes home from hospital or rehabilitation unit that the particular problems of such damaged people are highlighted, and there is sometimes massive disturbance to family relationships (Lezak, 1978).

What are the specific changes and difficulties experienced by brain-damaged people? Each individual has his/her own personality, abilities and approach to life. Therefore each person sees problems differently. All will experience some degree of loss and change. For severely brain-injured people, with both physical and intellectual damage, the loss may be devastating and the change total, and yet a patient may have only limited insight into this (Tyerman and Humphrey, 1986). For many, however, the changes may be subtle, and a person may present as physically quite well recovered. It is difficult for a family to cope with this. To outsiders or less involved relatives little actual change is apparent; for the spouse, parent, child or close relative, or possibly boy friend, girl friend, fiancé and fiancée there is a great difference in behaviour, and consequent interpersonal relationships. There is an essentially different quality to the personality and behaviour of those who have suffered moderate to severe brain damage, and this fact can sometimes elude the extended family or friends. It may also not

be apparent to the clinical team, with no pre-accident knowledge of the patient.

Consequently, when expectations of a full recovery, although
too high, are not attained, there is disappointment, resentment
and a sense of failure on the part of all involved. It can be that
the brain-injured patients are unaware of this; genuinely unable
to perceive change in themselves and puzzled by the reactions
of people they know. Pressure to continue living the usual
family life may confuse and upset the closest family members,
who are slowly beginning to realise that relationships have
changed to the point where this is no longer possible. The major
burden is beginning to be carried by the family (Weddell *et al.*,
1980).

THE SOCIAL EFFECTS OF BRAIN INJURY

Changes for the brain-injured person embrace a wide range of
factors:

(1) There is initial and possibly long-term physical disability.
    Previous strengths and capabilities have gone, and daily
    life may revolve around the progress to be gained and
    maintained in treatment programmes and activities. This
    is an acceptable area for the family to focus on at first,
    but the growing realisation of eventual physical depend-
    ence, for the patient and relatives, may be daunting.

(2) At the same time the severely brain-injured person has
    lost status. He or she may be unlikely to recover sufficiently
    to return to work. Only a small proportion do return to
    work, and often that has to be in a lesser capacity, or in
    sheltered workshops (Weddell *et al.*, 1980).

(3) Therefore there is loss of income, employment and
    consequently responsibility. Losses of this kind deeply
    affect family circumstances.

(4) Present accommodation may have to change if homes can
    no longer be afforded, or if accommodation does not meet
    the physical requirements of the patient.

(5) A wife may need to go back to work, and other carers
    have to come into the family unit to look after the patient
    and children. These can include in-laws, parents, sisters
    or friends, on a part-time or live-in basis. So there are

subtle shifts in family patterns, coupled with a loss of outside activity. People no longer relate in the same way, and there is a change of status within the family.

(6) The brain-injured patients will lose self-respect and may be depressed by their physical condition (Lewin *et al.*, 1979). The subsequent loss of friendships and contacts outside the family, combined with the loss of leisure activities (which produced these contacts) lead to a sense of isolation and loss.

The family experience similar loss. If the accident happened to the wage-earner the family also loses status and income. They have to make adjustments in the way they behave towards their brain-injured family member, and also in the structure of family life to accommodate him or her. Children have to suddenly become more adult, spouses become the main decision-maker (instead of being part of a couple or team), parents need to resume a parental role. All energies become concentrated on this one individual, with a grave loss to the other dependents and family members. There is less time for family social events and activities. Losing charge of his or her own affairs can lead to loneliness, isolation and depression, not only for the brain-injured person but also for the family — damaging family and social life.

Coupled with this set of problems the effects of perceptual, cognitive and personality changes in the head-injured individual may have wide-reaching effects. Serious memory problems affect relationships, causing anxiety and irritation for all involved, depriving the brain-injured person of shared memories. The patient may be severely impaired, forgetting immediate past events and being confused about chronological order. It is very difficult to sustain an emotional attachment to someone who has no recollection of your past and present together, and it requires strength and loving detachment for a partner to be able to do so. Brain injury can produce irritable, verbally and physically aggressive behaviour. As a result, lively children have to be quietened for fear of provoking temper and physical abuse. The family begin to tread warily, straining relationships. The injured person's needs may make him or her dominate in ways which vary from subtle to extreme. Many brain-injured people are very self-absorbed, not able to feel for others and needing a high degree of attention. They may be irresponsible, or so it seems to the family, behaving in casual and inappropriate ways which are greatly at odds with their previous personality. If they are restless and easily bored they may be asking for a greater degree of stimulus and attention than it is possible for relatives to give. However much the brain-injured person is loved by family and friends it may be increasingly difficult for him/her to be cared for when all the care and interest have to go one way, with little positive response or return of affection (Storey, 1981).

Whether these changes are being observed in hospital, rehabilitation centre or at home there is no doubt that after the initial crisis point is over there is a slowly dawning realisation that in the long term there are going to be changes which the family may find difficult to tolerate. At a time when there is a strong necessity for a grieving process for a lost personality the personification of that individual is still evident, confusing that mourning process. The injured person, though different, is very evidently alive, sometimes extremely demandingly so. The family is drained of strength and often lacks direction. Both the patient and the family may be denying reality, because the changes are too painful to acknowledge, whether in individual personality, family feelings or future ambitions. At a time when the clinical team are encouraged by physical and cognitive progress they may not be able to recognise the family dilemma (Lewin *et al.*, 1979; Lezak, 1978; Livingston, 1986a).

THE SOCIAL WORK ROLE

The social worker is presented with some of the same problems as the family. It is not possible for the social worker to establish any meaningful relationship with the brain-injured patient during the coma and post-traumatic amnesia stage. In the latter each new contact is of the moment, and not usually remembered. Even in the later stages of recovery the social worker will have difficulty in establishing a counselling relationship with a person who has, through no fault of his/her own, lack of insight; who can be egocentric and facetious; who is poorly motivated towards improvement and change, and who is locked into obsessional ideas. The feeling that to confront the patient with such factors is cruel can be a complicating factor, but none the less the social worker, unlike the family, can be objective and can put forward a more balanced perspective of the difficulties experienced and likely outcome for the family. With specialised knowledge and experience the social worker can reassure the family that certain stages can be expected both in their own and the families' emotional and physical recovery, and that they can expect support and guidance.

Discharging the brain-injured person home into the community should involve a very clear and definite continuation of support, guidance and advice for the patient and the family. It may be that visits to the hospital or clinic have diminished and the responsibility for support comes best from community-based occupational, speech and physiotherapists and social workers. The hospital social worker should ensure that the patient and family do not feel abandoned on the discharge of the patient home. If possible the home-based social worker should visit patient and family prior to discharge, or the hospital social worker should continue visiting at home until a positive transfer of responsibility is achieved. Unlike some rehabilitation processes the problems will intensify when the family is reunited, and this is a vital time for continuing professional counselling, not just with legal, financial and practical concerns, but to meet both current and future emotional needs of the family. As Lezak (1978) has stated, the family are going to need information and guidance even though they are very likely to be unwilling to accept it at this stage. The social worker must try to establish an honest and supportive relationship in preparation for the inevitable difficulties ahead. All possible action, whether statutory or voluntary, should be provided to support the brain-injured person and the family once the acute treatment and rehabilitation process is over, because recovery may continue for several years.

Professional counselling is needed, in addition to the comfort, friendship and advice offered by relatives and friends. The spouse, parent or child and other relatives need someone to whom it is 'safe' to talk, who has no vested emotional interests in the situation. They will need to express negative as well as positive thoughts. They will have fears and anxieties, resentments and difficulties. Previously they shared problems with the brain-injured person, but now that close relationship has gone. The wider group of family and friends may not want, or be able, to hear the negative feelings the close relatives need to express, as it conflicts with their own needs and reactions. For the family the brain-injured person needs to be integrated and accepted in a new way, and this may be unacceptable to those not living closely with the problem.

If disturbance is severe as a result of the loss of the brain-injured person's previous role within the family there may be a need for family or individual therapy, perhaps conjointly with a psychiatrist or psychologist. Clinical treatment may be needed for a while in cases of anxiety and depression (Livingston, 1986a). Medication should not be given in isolation, and in some instances the need for this may be ameliorated by consistent support from a social worker perceived as being accessible and helpful, to whom feelings can be safely ventilated.

The social worker must be able to accept feelings of anger and resentment from patients and relatives, to support those in distress and despair, and to act on behalf of both patient and family. This is important in preparation for a later stage when it becomes necessary, for the family's emotional health and well-being, to lay down guidelines for new responsibilities and roles within the family. If the social worker is seen as being equally committed to both 'sides' it is easier for the family not to view any future rearrangement to their family unit structure and function as being disloyal to the brain-injured family member. This may reduce the guilt often felt when the family have to, in a sense, ignore the brain-injured person's stated wishes for themselves, in favour of a plan which accommodates all the family's needs, as well as their own. The social worker acts as a moderator, embracing all the viewpoints expressed, but with necessary detachment and objectivity, plans for and protects the welfare of the whole family.

One so often hears described the need for the family's involvement in the brain-injured person's rehabilitation. Their loss, however, is equally acute, or possibly (because of the long-term responsibilities involved) more acute than that of the brain-injured person. The clinical team needs to support and understand the family reaction, and even be prepared for the possible disintegration of the family. During counselling the social worker should allow for all kinds of future arrangements to be discussed, as part of the family's rehabilitation. Paradoxically, allowing the family to contemplate separation or divorce may have the effect of changing or improving the relationship between the brain-injured person and the relatives.

Where families are able and prepared to be involved in rehabilitation they can be encouraged to do so. However, there should not be too heavy an emphasis on this, as each family is unique, and coping skills will vary tremendously. If separation occurs, preparation and counselling may enable it to happen in an atmosphere of decreased tension, and continued friendships, where the spouse in particular is able to regard himself or herself as remaining the 'best friend' of the brain-injured person, without having to pretend an emotional depth of relationship which is no longer present.

Perhaps the most sensitive and difficult area to treat in counselling of spouses is sexual relationships. 'It's like making love to a stranger' was the title of a talk given by Anne Needham to Headway London Conference in 1986, and this phrase encapsulates the feelings of many spouses of the brain-injured. The problems are varied, and it can be some time before spouses are prepared to talk about altered sexual relations. Brain-injured spouses may become sexually in-appropriate and excessively demanding, to the embarrassment and dismay of their partner. They may be flirtatious and sexually demonstrative towards other people, even proposition-ing complete strangers. Conversely, where a couple had a close and loving relationship the injured partner may show no sexual interest, and this unemotional or distant response may be hurtful. A change in personality or behaviour may mean the non-injured partner is no longer able to respond emotionally or sexually to a previously well-loved spouse, causing that spouse, now brain-injured, sadness or irritation.

The injured person may display jealousy or anger in a way that limits the non-injured partner's normal daily routine in a very difficult way. It is especially important that the married or other close partners receive counselling and advice with, above all, understanding, to lessen guilt and anxiety felt about the loss of sexual response. Though not necessarily separating, the couple's relationship may change into one of loving friendship rather than intimacy. This is more easily achieved if the brain-injured person's libido is diminished (Lezak, 1978) rather than in the presence of hypersexuality. The brain-injured person may be less able to come to terms with the change of response, where the latter exists, and will need ongoing advice and help from the clinical team, particularly in dealing with sexual frustration, which in itself can cause behavioural problems.

THE EXPERIENCE OF READJUSTMENT

Each family situation is unique, and not all follow the same pattern, but there are enough similarities to form the basis for general expectations of reactions and strategies.

The young wife

Very young marriages often cannot cope with the stress imposed by changes in personality, emotional response and physical abilities of the brain-injured partner. A wife with young children may feel she had had her partner returned to her, after injury and rehabilitation, as another child of the family. However, this 'child' can be more irritable and aggressive than other children, unable to monitor his own behaviour. He may become demanding and attention-seeking, vying with his own children for his wife's interest. She, instead of having a partner with whom to share family life and the children's upbringing, has additional worry with less support than before. The family unit becomes isolated, especially if the family has to move and is no longer near friends and family.

Wives with teenage children

A wife with more years of marriage behind her, with teenage children, may react to the experience of living with a brain-damaged partner in a different way. She may have a strong and happy marriage, which has weathered other difficulties. She may feel strength and commitment to the partner because of the good previous marital relationship. Her children are more actual support to her than her husband, and despite difficulties she may experience more positive factors in family life, because they are able to discuss things with her and take a more adult role in mutually sharing grief and loss.

Teenagers have to take on adult roles, and for boys this can present special problems when the father returns home and expects to reassume an authoritative role. Teenagers change a great deal in a few years, and because of this may find their father cannot cope with their progress, competing with them

175

and trying to re-establish a superior and controlling position (Lezak, 1978).

Marriage of older partners

It would appear that wives in longer-lasting marriages may be able to adapt to living with a brain-injured husband, unless there are problem behaviours such as possessive and obsessional characteristics (Lezak, 1978). Usually partners would find it difficult to contemplate separation or divorce after a previously long and affectionate marriage. Physical disability appears to be a more acceptable problem to be faced than the subtle personality changes brought about by brain damage, and this is not peculiar to older partners.

The brain-injured woman

There is less available information about the family circumstances where young women are injured, as the ratio of women to men to suffer brain damage is one in three. In the case of young and newly married women experience would predict that these marriages do not survive the period of initial hospitalisation and rehabilitation, so that young married women once again become the responsibility of their parents.

The extended family

Grandparents or grandchildren of brain-injured individuals are often accepting of differences in behaviour and, it seems, find ways of assisting and supporting their relatives. Just as is usual in family life, the relationship between grandparent and grandchild is often more relaxed, one step removed from the emotional depth and interaction between parent and child, and this distance is helpful.

The single person

Accidents frequently happen to young people who are not in

relationships, to single parents and those who are widowed and divorced. For such isolated brain-injured people an attachment forms to the rehabilitation team, rather than other patients, as the sense of identification is stronger.

Some may deliberately delay their own progress and resort to more acting-out behaviour to demonstrate they are not willing or ready to leave the rehabilitation unit.

THE FAMILY AND THE REHABILITATION TEAM

A rehabilitation team should establish contact with family and friends throughout treatment so that plans can be formulated together for the brain-injured person's care on discharge from the unit.

It is very important for clinical and rehabilitation teams not to be judgemental about relatives at any stage. It is easy to perceive a family as being difficult if they seem either over-involved or uncooperative. The family may be very disillusioned by what they see as previous failures in treatment and rehabilitation, or depressed by slow or negligible progress. They may not believe, or may not be able to allow themselves to believe, that any new rehabilitative approach may achieve a positive result. They may in fact be afraid to hope. The results of an accident and subsequent brain damage can have profound effects on previously ordinary family relationships, and families may not be able to present themselves well when under severe stress. Families, shocked and devastated by what has happened to their relative, may have developed their own coping strategies. They may be critical about the patient's physical care whilst in rehabilitation, finding fault and getting into conflict with the team (McLaughlin and Schaffer, 1985).

The family may still be hoping and fighting for a full recovery, and may view anything less as a failure. All these roles are hard to relinquish and one should be careful, as a rehabilitation team, to help the family to understand and accept realistic hopes for future progress (Birley and Hudson, 1983). Sometimes when a patient appears to an enthusiastic team to be making progress it is hard when a family is apparently not encouraging or realistic, perhaps because the improvement is not as much as they hoped for.

THE SOCIAL WORKER IN THE REHABILITATION TEAM

In some ways the social worker is well placed to translate the aims and goals of the treatment team to the relatives, and vice-versa, though hopefully the need for this role should diminish as the family get to know and have more confidence in the rehabilitation unit.

When their brain-injured relative is admitted to a rehabilitation unit the family can relax — perhaps for the first time since the crisis period. Partners, other relatives and friends can begin to examine in depth their own feelings and fears about their own reactions, and their future. The social worker should be prepared for the fact that for some families the grieving process is continuing. It may be further thrown into conflict when, during rehabilitation, the brain-injured person is being helped to control difficult behaviour, is no longer sedated and is redeveloping his or her personality and character. Changes are made which influence the way in which brain-injured people are viewed by their families. Usually the increased mobility and physical independence lessen the family burden, but can have aspects which are frightening. The family members need to feel involved and have reasonable access to the whole treatment team, as well as the social worker. The family need information on progress and advice on management, especially if their relative is beginning to spend some time at home. This is most easily arranged at small family sessions with team members, but can also involve family members attending some therapy sessions. At the same time one may also need to encourage the family to take time off from their problems, to take holidays, find recreational activities, to be free from responsibilities and anxieties for even brief periods, perhaps for the first time in years.

Obviously the social worker's other main tasks, as well as counselling and the amassing of social and family histories, is to plan for residential care after discharge, employment or some reasonable daily activity where possible, and good follow-up. The social worker needs the expertise of the rehabilitation team, as well as the resources of statutory and voluntary agencies, to achieve the best possible outcome for the brain-injured individuals, in the light of their own unique personality, life experience and family relationships.

PLANNING FOR FUTURE NEEDS

It is unfortunate that specialist rehabilitation units tend to have large catchment areas, and it may only be possible to offer a limited after-care service. It is therefore necessary to begin to make arrangements well before the patient leaves hospital. Ideally one should be able to work with agencies in the patient's home area throughout the rehabilitation period. Home-based social workers should attend unit reviews and assessments, together with the family. They will begin to establish relationships with the brain-injured person and their families when decisions are being made as to the future; whether they are going to live with their families or are going to live in hostels, group homes, or homes of their own.

If a court case and compensation settlement is anticipated the social worker can often assist the family solicitors, using past and present experience to anticipate likely costs involved in future care. There is very little specialist residential accommodation available for the brain-injured. Unless they can be cared for by family members there is little chance of finding appropriate residential circumstances. Often all that is available in the home area is a mental handicap hospital. Not surprisingly, individuals and their families do not find this acceptable. Seeing such alternatives does not enable families to separate without guilt, even though it might be in the best interests of all that they should do so, because there is no ideal facility in which the brain-injured person can live happily, and can be seen by the family to be properly cared for.

Hopefully, with the increasing emphasis on community care — in both the United States and the United Kingdom — large hospitals and residential communities for mentally handicapped people, however good, will not be seen as the answer to the needs of those with brain injury. They need small residential units with an emphasis on a mixture of structure, activity and recreation in a homelike atmosphere. They would need a high staff ratio and specially trained staff able to accept occasionally difficult behaviour. Despite the need for some supervision of daily activities there should also be an emphasis on choice and freedom of initiative to as great a degree as possible. In the United States the transitional living facility may partially fulfil this role.

LIVING INDEPENDENTLY

In the absence of such ideal facilities it has been possible in specially selected cases to establish brain-injured people in homes of their own. Many individuals do have quite substantial damages, awarded by the courts, in compensation for their injuries. Such cases can take years to settle, but solicitors can often obtain interim payments, against future settlements, to provide for treatment and care. If a brain-injured person has sufficient funds a suitable house can be purchased, adapted, equipped and furnished. Some individuals are occasionally able to live alone with support from community services; others need live-in carers. For the severely brain-injured who have made a reasonable recovery with only minimal behavioural problems it is necessary to explore the possibility of home-based schemes almost as a matter of choice.

Where a decision has had to be made that the brain-injured person is not going to live with parent or spouse and children, and if provision for independent housing can be made because of compensation settlement, then thought has to be given to the kind of person who is going to be employed as companion and care-giver. There are some schemes in the United Kingdom organised by Social Services, to employ, provide and supervise residential social workers to live with and support vulnerable individuals in homes of their own. Such schemes undertake to make the vulnerable person as fully participant in normal society as possible.

Experience has shown that for one person, without relief, to look after a brain-injured person for months on end, leads inevitably to a deterioration in the relationship and unendurable stress for the carer. This is particularly so with relatives where the greater the magnitude of behavioural and personality change in the patient the higher the stress level. The situation does not improve with time (Brooks *et al.*, 1986).

One useful and successful solution has been to engage the services of agencies who supply experienced companions and almost by a system of trial-and-error establish a nucleus of companions for each patient who comes on a monthly rota basis. They should be carefully chosen, either by the family or together with the social worker, and the placements will, initially at least, involve some supervision to ensure that the brain-injured client and the companion are well-suited and the carers understand their role and can carry it out. Care-givers need to be compassionate but able to be firm, providing a basic structure and routine to daily life, but also able to be flexible, ensuring the brain-injured persons have as much choice as possible about the way they spend their time and lives.

Because these companions come from private agencies it would protect the interests, and special needs, of the brain-injured person if a social worker could supervise such arrangements.

Employing live-in companions in houses specially purchased and adapted may seem expensive, but once established these do not necessarily cost more than accommodation in residential hostels or communities or hospitals. Such schemes may, if properly staffed and supervised, give independence of lifestyle.

CONCLUSION

One family in 300 (in the United Kingdom) has a member with persisting disability after head injury, and this is apt to cause secondary morbidity in other family members, sometimes resulting in permanent disruption of relationships (*Lancet*, 1983).

It should not be forgotten that for most brain-injured people their problems are the result of unanticipated and sudden circumstances which have changed their lives. They have special problems physically and cognitively. In spite of possibly normal intelligence they may be unable to express themselves as they would wish, or may misperceive information given to them. They may be unable to read and write because of their perceptual or learning difficulties. They may be frustrated or depressed, angry or withdrawn, with all the attendant problems associated with mood changes. Brain dysfunction can influence the individual's present relationships and impair the development of new ones. Successful emotional recovery usually requires uncomplicated communication and reasonable insight, which is often not present. The brain-injured person may not be able to express emotions normally (Luria, 1972). Emotions may be expressed in childish or over-demonstrative ways, causing grief and embarrassment to the family.

Despite all their problems most brain-injured people are working together with their rehabilitation therapists in determined ways to achieve maximum recovery. The family also faces unique problems in respect of a brain-injured relative. The magazine *Headway News*, published in the United Kingdom by the National Head Injuries Association, describes the personal struggles and experiences of the brain-injured and their families and therapists in a moving and salutary way. It is true that as yet only Headway and a few specialist rehabilitation centres assist and support the brain-injured and their relatives. It has been suggested in this chapter that without the provision of proper community resources brain-injured persons may not be able to move on from hospital and, even if they do so, may create unmanageable stress and burden to their relatives. There is now documented knowledge and research into the effect and treatment of brain injury both for the individual and family. Counselling itself will help (Lezak, 1978), but without practical resources the long-term outcome for those who have suffered brain injury is going to depend on where the individual lives, and whether or not any private or voluntary services can be utilised to provide a solution to what is very often a devastating and socially limiting injury. From the acute stage, through to the rehabilitation and return to the community, patients and their relatives deserve maximum support and services which cater creatively and realistically to their very special needs.

10

The Application of a Behavioural Model in Rehabilitation

Ian Fussey, with John Cumberpatch and Claire Grant

Many of the chapters in this book contain practical approaches to rehabilitation along with some of the theoretical considerations underlying their use. Some of the techniques described are highly specialised, and there may be readers who, working in some areas of brain injury, feel that the techniques portrayed belong in specialist units. While it may have to be accepted that some forms of rehabilitation require special settings, this chapter aims to give an outline of the basic requirements of a team approach to rehabilitation using a behavioural model.

With the recognition of certain constraints, rehabilitation staff in a variety of settings can apply a behavioural model. However, the application of this kind of model does have costs. Working with the brain-injured adult can at times be stressful and unrewarding. The application of a behavioural model requires a certain shift in professional attitude, which can itself be stressful. Even so, the benefits to the patient may be considered to outweigh the costs to the rehabilitation team.

The rehabilitation team will be discussed in terms of the way rehabilitation services are provided. A 'users' guide' to techniques of behaviour management will be presented, with reference to the constraints imposed by the variety of settings of brain injury rehabilitation.

THE REHABILITATION TEAM

Brain-injured adults often receive rehabilitation from a range of professionals working independently; occupational therapists, speech therapists, physiotherapists and so forth. The term 'multidisciplinary team' has been used to describe this situation. The term implies that a group of professionals are working together towards a defined goal but, unfortunately, words are not necessarily deeds. Most readers of this book will be professionals of one form or another and we are all aware that we each secretly believe that our discipline has the most to offer. Therefore the members of multidisciplinary teams may all be doing what they think is appropriate for the patient's needs, but it may not be coordinated in a common goal. Whatever the 'team' is called, be it interdisciplinary or transdisciplinary, it does not really matter, providing a rehabilitation team works together.

The behavioural model, which considers functional goals rather than therapist-generated targets, requires that the team work together in such a way that each individual therapist can understand how his or her professional input can be linked to that of their colleagues of other disciplines. While this requires a considerable degree of communication it may also lead to the need for therapists to 'blur' their role boundaries in order to fulfil the patient's needs.

Blurring of professional roles

Role blurring is known to be stressful in most work settings. Most professionals spend a considerable part of their early career developing a professional identity. However, those working with the brain-injured need not lose their professional identity in order to belong to such a rehabilitation team; on the contrary each professional brings to the team his or her own particular professional strengths.

One of the best ways for a rehabilitation team to develop a group identity is to ensure good communication between all team members. Ideally this should include all those who come into contact with the patient, in order that an overall treatment plan can be carried out consistently, especially where specific behaviour management is included. The task of learning new skills is difficult enough for the brain-injured patient, but confusion between therapists as to the aims and methods of achieving such learning will produce more problems.

This book has emphasised the need for consistency. Communication between team members can be of a high standard, but staff can rotate between different units or wards, causing possible problems with consistency. The ideal situation would be one of unit-based staffing. An important role is potentially available for nursing staff. It is they who are with the patient 24 hours a day and, with good communication between nursing shifts, it is desirable for them to assume responsibility for overall day-to-day programme management. Frequent changes of staff are therefore not only confusing where patients are concerned, but also increase the problems of implementing behavioural management programmes. This arises partly because of the difficulty in training new staff quickly enough to avoid them inappropriately reinforcing undesirable behaviours.

Unfortunately we do not live in an ideal world. Most of those working in rehabilitation settings will, at one time or another, have questioned the motives of those who manage the treatment facilities. One begins to wonder whether staff allocations are planned for the convenience of administrators or the benefit of patients. The fact remains that new staff will have to be incorporated into the treatment team from time to time, to cover vacation or sickness absence.

The need for adequate staff training is covered in Chapter 3 in regard to the management of behavioural disorders, but education is also important if a team approach to brain injury rehabilitation is to be produced. If it is accepted that an interactional rehabilitation approach aimed at functional goals is the treatment of choice, then a closer working relationship between therapists is required. While a greater understanding of the methods of therapists of different disciplines can be an advantage, it may also lead to colleagues coming up with new ideas as to how one may actually treat the patient. For many professionals this can be a daunting prospect. However, it must be remembered that such new ideas can be of benefit to the patient, and professional ego must take second place. Even so, if this is education, then it will be seen that to preserve team harmony it should proceed in a constructive manner.

It should not be too difficult to set up a reasonably thorough system of staff education, using a form of in-service training based upon individual therapists training other disciplines in the rudiments of their skills. Additionally, to deal with new staff, one of us (I.F.) found it useful to develop a basic information booklet, containing a broad outline of the aims and methods of the rehabilitation unit and a description of the behaviour management procedures (in the USA called a treatment protocol). Specific behaviour management techniques will be presented later in this chapter, but many rehabilitation units will have access to a psychology department from whence advice can be sought.

BEHAVIOURAL MANAGEMENT: A USERS' GUIDE

The primary task in behavioural management is assessment. If performed correctly this allows for a quantitative evaluation of the current state of behaviour or skills level and will facilitate an objective view of improvement (or lack of improvement). Assessment should include both excesses and deficits of the behaviour or skill measured, but should also extend beyond the actual behaviour to consider the circumstances in which the behaviour takes place. If one takes into account both the antecedent and the consequence of the behaviour, then what is measured is a 'behavioural event'. Knowledge of the behavioural event allows for the behaviour or skill to be modified by changing the antecedent or the consequence of the behaviour, thus the A–B–C recording of behaviour (see Table 10.1). With the information gained from this recording, in the case presented in Table 10.1, the patient hitting therapist and avoiding therapy, it is possible to change either the antecedent (another therapist, perhaps), or change the consequences so that aggression is not successful in avoiding therapy (Cuvo and Davis, 1983).

The use of the A–B–C recording will also show whether a behaviour or skill can be performed in one setting or circumstance rather than another which, unless known, can prevent an understanding of the patient's true level of functioning

Table 10.1: The A–B–C record

Antecedent
Patient has been brought down to physiotherapy in a wheelchair. Patient is asked to remove wheelchair armrests and swing aside footrests prior to transferring to the bed.
Behaviour
Patient begins shouting and swearing at staff. He refuses to cooperate and attempts to be physically aggressive.
Consequence
Therapist calls the patient's ward to have a nurse come and remove the patient. The patient avoids therapy.

(Goldstein and Ruthven, 1983). What is necessary is an analysis of the patient's ability to carry out a task in a range of settings. It seems rather a waste of time to devote so much energy to devising tests said to be similar to real-life tasks when one can assess the patient in a real-life situation.

It is often suggested that to focus on a behavioural model is to deny the existence of thoughts and feelings. A more realistic interpretation is that thoughts and feelings are not given as much salience in a behavioural approach as in other treatment approaches. A behavioural event is a behavioural event, regardless of the emotional state of the individual, although the emotional state of the individual can be inferred from observable behaviour and could then be considered as a possible antecedent. We usually infer 'happy' from the behaviour of smiling, and 'depressed' from decreased motor activity. What is important in assessment is to define the behaviour or skill in such a way that all team members can agree on its occurrence or non-occurrence. The problem with emotional states, or vague terms such as 'getting better', is that they are liable to subjective interpretation and can therefore invalidate measurements. Even so, a behavioural approach does not deny the individual's thoughts and feelings and the right to express them within socially acceptable limits.

Functional assessment

Most professionals working with the brain-injured have methods of assessment — some formal, some informal, the latter often depending on personal experience. The problem with many of these assessments is that they give little indication of the problems faced by the patient in a natural setting. The results are often difficult to interpret by other disciplines, so while such formal assessments can be useful in giving an academic perspective on the patient's problems within specific areas, there is obviously a need for functionally based assessment of skills and disabilities.

This can be done simply by observing the patient in a variety of settings — Is performance variable? Are there certain settings that cause a change in performance? Are these person-specific, i.e. is performance better with one therapist than another? From this it is possible to highlight a number of problem areas, perhaps combining results from more formal assessment. Only following full assessment is sufficient information available to begin to plan treatment approaches, taking into account the likely future environment of the patient.

Deciding on priorities

In the case of severe brain injury it is not always possible, or even advisable, to try to work on all problems simultaneously. It is necessary for the treatment team to decide on priorities. Deciding on the first problem or set of problems can be difficult if little or no communication exists between therapy disciplines. For example the speech therapist may see communication problems as a priority, whereas the physiotherapist may see 'his or her' area of mobility as the main problem. It should not be forgotten that the priorities to be considered foremost are those that will maximally assist the patient's rehabilitation. For example, to initially consider mobility may improve posture and actually increase social contact for the patient, thus allowing for the increased chance of practice of communication skills. It should be obvious that in the best interests of the patient the hierarchy of priorities for rehabilitation should be discussed by the full treatment team and, wherever possible, the patient and his or her family. Naturally, priorities will also depend upon practical matters such as staff availability, and the interrelatedness and urgency of problems.

Functional analysis and setting targets

This requires reducing the problem to its component parts, to facilitate learning of what may be a complex skill or behaviour. Having established the current baseline of the targeted behaviour it is at this point, before therapy commences, that it is possible to set targets for change. Like behaviours or skills, targets should be tangible and clear to all concerned, not least the patient. If the targets are reasonable and likely to be obtained then they can enhance motivation for patient and therapist by charting recovery in a way that is readily apparent. Given that in some cases recovery of skills following brain injury can be slow, it can sometimes be disheartening for patient and therapist when little apparent progress is made; setting targets makes small increments of improvement, which might otherwise go unnoticed, more visible.

There are a number of techniques used to manage problem behaviours or to assist in the learning or relearning of new behaviours or skills. A recent review of research indicates an increasing trend towards using behaviour therapy with brain-injured individuals (Horton and Miller, 1985). The principles of reinforcement or reward have been covered in Chapter 3 and will not be considered here, although there is an important general principle to remember, which is, whenever possible, to reward the occurrence of appropriate or desired behaviour, rather than penalise the patient in some way for inappropriate or undesirable behaviour. This makes for a far more positive attitude on the part of the therapy staff, and also avoids ethical problems. If it is feasible, therefore, one's motto should be to reinforce all desirable behaviours and strenuously ignore all inappropriate behaviours.

Notwithstanding this advice it may be necessary, due to the extreme nature of the undesirable behaviour, to use more drastic forms of management. These will be discussed below, although their use should be restricted to situations where the problem behaviour is likely to lead to harm to the patient from self-injurious behaviour (Eames and Wood, 1985a). It is important that all staff should understand the principles underlying such approaches and accept their use (see Wood and Eames, 1981).

Specific techniques of behaviour management

Time-out

In specialist behavioural units this procedure may involve taking the patient to a locked, bare room, where he/she remains under close, though discreet, observation, for a period of two to five minutes. Often used following episodes of physical aggression it is designed to remove patients from the reinforcement of the results of their actions, such as the attention they might receive (Ullmann and Krasner, 1969). At a practical level this technique gives all staff a positive response to situations that could be threatening, and escalate out of control without this well-defined response to aggression.

As such a room is not always available on most rehabilitation units, therapy staff can place patients into a corridor, or at the other end of the room if it is safe to do so. As a last resort, if the patient cannot be moved, the therapist may simply walk away from the patient, but return within two minutes, acting as if nothing had happened (a difficult task if one has been struck). This is necessary to deny the patient the gratification of knowing he has caused harm or discomfort. This form of time-out can be refined, as in the next technique.

TOOTS (time-out-on-the-spot)

This procedure involves not reinforcing or rewarding the patient for inappropriate behaviour. This can be done in two ways. One method is to not pay attention to the individual on the production of inappropriate behaviour for a brief period of 20 seconds by, for example, moving away or talking to someone else.

A second way is for the therapist to continue to pay attention to the patient but to ignore the inappropriate behaviour. The latter method is most suitable when a therapy activity is proceeding and should not be interrupted. This approach would be exemplified by a walking programme:

> *Therapist*: 'Grasp the walking frame and move on the instruction, Push, Step, Shift. Push the frame, one step, then shift your weight.'
> *Patient* (shouting): 'Is this what you want, you stinking cow?'
> *Therapist*: 'Push, Step, Shift.'
> *Patient*: 'Bloody whore!'
> *Therapist*: 'That was a good step, let's try again.'

Note how the therapist ignores the patient's inappropriate verbalisation and concentrates on the goal of teaching the patient how to walk.

Shaping

It is not always possible to reinforce new desirable behaviours, because in many cases the desired response may never occur. Shaping refers to the reinforcement of small steps or closer and closer approximations to the desired behaviour. For example, J.B.R. (described elsewhere in this volume) would pace around the unit in a very agitated state during tea and coffee breaks.

The goal was to encourage him to sit with others and engage in appropriate conversation. Initially J.B.R. was rewarded for just staying in the room with everybody else, with attention, praise and a tangible reinforcer. Later he was only reinforced when he was sitting down, and still later only reinforced for sitting quietly or in socially appropriate conversation.

As the initial approximation is performed consistently, the criterion for reinforcement is altered slightly so that the next response resembles the final goal more closely than did the previous response. This continues until the final goal is achieved (Craighead *et al.*, 1976).

Modelling

This term generally implies social imitation in the context of behaviour management. This process is the means by which new responses are acquired, reinforced or extinguished at a distance, through observation of the behaviour of others. A large proportion of our behavioural repertoire is developed in this way, not through experience, but through observing others in particular circumstances and how they fare as a consequence (Sheldon, 1982).

Modelling can therefore be a process by which the brain-injured patients can learn new skills in many areas of deficiency. It therefore follows that all personnel in contact with the brain-injured patient are potential models. It should be remembered that the phrase 'Do as I say, not as I do' has no relevance here. If therapy staff expect patients to behave appropriately then they too should behave appropriately. Social skills and posture are areas of particular relevance.

Prompting

Events that help initiate a behaviour are called prompts. If the prompt produced a targeted behaviour (or an approximation) then that behaviour can be reinforced. As a general rule, when a prompt consistently precedes reinforcement of a response, then that prompt becomes a discriminant stimulus (see below) and can effectively control behaviour (Craighead *et al.*, 1976).

Using a prompt can speed the learning of new behaviours. Therapists can facilitate the learning of new skills by either physical or verbal prompts. Physical prompts can include physically guiding the required behaviour. Verbal prompts involve instructing in the production of the required behaviour.

Once the behaviour or new skill is developed then the prompts should no longer be necessary. Once the final goal is achieved it is necessary to reduce the prompting, which is artificial, and allow the behaviour to be sustained independently. The process of reducing prompts is known as fading. Fade the prompt too early and the response may diminish. Prompts should be faded gradually, and the prompts that will be the first to be faded are those where an environmental cue takes its place, for example, in the prompted sequence 'wash, rinse, dry', the prompts 'rinse' and 'dry' would become redundant before the 'wash' prompt, because being wet acts as a cue to rinsing and drying.

Discriminant learning

Discriminant learning, as used in this context, is a term borrowed and adapted from animal learning experiments. In helping the brain-injured patient to learn new skills or behaviours it is important that they are assisted to discriminate between behaviours that have positive outcome and those that have a negative outcome. For example, when reinforcement is given for a behaviour it is important to make clear to the patient the reason for the reinforcement, as in 'Well done, it's really good to see you sitting so well!' The reinforcement is strongly linked to the behaviour, which will enhance learning. The principle is equally important when applying a modification of a time-out programme in a case of excessive physical contact or inappropriate touching. As the patient is removed from the setting, a therapist can say 'Touch' in a matter-of-fact, unemotional tone, and thus link the behaviour of excessive touching with the negative consequences of time out with the discriminant stimulus of 'Touch'.

Other behavioural techniques are most suitably used with specific behaviour disorders although, as mentioned previously, some of these should be reserved for 'last resort' situations when the behaviour disorder is especially severe. In general these techniques — such as over-correction, massed practice and aversive techniques such as the use of ammonia vapour — are both time-consuming to administer and have limited value in the majority of the brain-injured population. In any event their use should always be supervised by an experienced clinical psychologist.

Most behavioural techniques are simply the commonsense application of a number of rules. Within this heading it should not be forgotten that one of the simplest behavioural techniques at the disposal of therapists is practice.

While these techniques are designed to facilitate the learning of new skills and behaviours, it is hoped that these skills will be retained by the patient and applied in new settings. The true test of learning is generalisation of a learned skill to a completely unfamiliar environment.

WHY BEHAVIOURAL MANAGEMENT MAY FAIL

Consistency

A lack of staff consistency can seriously jeopardise the success of behavioural management. Failure to consistently reinforce appropriate behaviour or skills, or respond to inappropriate behaviour, will equally prevent effective learning. *Remedy*: clear goals and targets understood by the whole treatment team.

Communication

Poor communication between team members will adversely affect consistency. The aim should be to have all members of the treatment team aware of their colleagues' roles and how their own contribution relates to the overall approach. In carrying out a behavioural approach it may be that certain team members disagree with an adopted technique for managing disturbed behaviour. It is better that such disagreements are voiced openly, rather than covertly disrupting the consistency of approach. Team members must feel able to voice their views. *Remedy*: regular team meetings that allow for discussion, in an atmosphere of trust within the team.

Flexibility

The behavioural model relies on approaches that are functional and designed to fit the patient's needs, rather than a textbook's guidelines. Flexibility is needed to step out of one's professional role. *Remedy*: put the need of the patient first.

Institutional constraints

It may be that this model is inappropriate because of constraints beyond the power of the team to change. There could be a lack of available resources. *Remedy*: keep fighting the system and don't give up hope!

Learning constraints

It may have to be accepted that some patients, because of their injury, will reach the limits of their learning before many functional gains have been made and, despite the strenuous efforts of the team, no more improvements can be made. At this point perhaps the best that can be done is to secure a placement for the patient that gives the best quality of life compatible with functional ability. It is necessary to accept that with limited resources it is not cost-effective to continue attempts at rehabilitation beyond the point where learning is not demonstrated.

CONCLUSION

It will be clear to anyone working in the field of brain injury rehabilitation that this approach places more pressure upon staff in an already stressful area. This type of work, when considered from an organisational perspective, is potentially stressful. Interacting with patients and colleagues may be difficult. Rehabilitation is usually carried out in an organisation with an hierarchical structure, which poses pressures, in most cases from above and below, depending on one's seniority in the organisation. And, of course, therapists are only human, with their individual problems outside of the work environment.

It may appear that many of the factors of the behavioural approach to brain injury rehabilitation seem to exacerbate those areas of work practice that we already know to be stressful. It is suggested that the advantages gained, in terms of job satisfaction at demonstrable achievements, will more than compensate. This has attempted to be a practical look at implementing programmes of rehabilitation. No doubt some problems in implementation have been missed, but it is left to individual therapists working as a team to solve those problems, in the most advantageous way for their needs.

11

The Future of Brain Injury Rehabilitation

Ian Fussey and Gordon Muir Giles

This book presents a practical approach to brain injury rehabilitation for professionals. Families of brain-injured patients may also find the information helpful. In spite of providing a practical guide it has been our intention to incorporate the approach within a behavioural model or framework. It is now necessary to consider the future developments of brain injury rehabilitation.

Work is continuing in laboratories to find methods of assisting brain tissue regeneration, or preventing the degeneration of tissue not destroyed by trauma, but which frequently dies soon thereafter (Freed *et al.*, 1985). While these techniques could hold great promise for the future, practical rehabilitation is required at present.

The previous chapters have argued for the adoption of a coherent model of rehabilitation by all therapy staff. Within the United Kingdom, patient management is the notional responsibility of medical consultants of various specialties who, with a number of exceptions, have little day-to-day contact with the patient. They are expected to take a leading role in the management of their patients. In practice, however, this is delegated to therapy staff, who lack a coordinated approach. Therefore planning of treatment at best lacks detail and at the worst is fragmentary. If the behavioural model is adopted it is even more important to have a unified approach with adequate day-to-day direction. The system crucially depends on consistency and effective communication. In the United States there exists a system known as case management. Case managers take responsibility for the management of individual patient care and ensure that there is a coordinated approach. This role could be fulfilled by a clinical coordinator, who could be a member of any of the professional therapy disciplines involved in brain injury rehabilitation. A further development would be to extend the role of the clinical coordinator to that of a case coordinator, working for an individual brain-injured patient and not affiliated to any one unit. This 'higher-level' coordinator could manage the patient's needs from injury onwards.

Not only does the unified management approach need to be adopted at the unit or ward level, but this also requires a change in policy at a higher administrative level. Jennett (1982) has claimed that greater resources are required to meet the needs of the brain-injured adult. To effectively change the structure of service provision for the brain-injured, the policy-makers at higher levels in health service management must be made aware of both current and future needs. Unfortunately considerable financial allocation is required to create even the minimal acceptable level of care.

The development of a consistent approach within a rehabilitation team is an admirable goal. Until a consensus can be reached as to the style and level of rehabilitation provision, resources for its implementation are not likely to be forthcoming. Brain injury rehabilitation will be governed to some extent by constraints beyond the team's power to change, such as environmental or financial constraints. This may prevent certain units from being able to cope with severe behaviour disorder arising from brain injury, or from adequately integrating the patient into the community. This will realistically be left to specialist units. There is, however, no reason why the move towards functional assessment and rehabilitation should not proceed.

Brain injury rehabilitation is a highly specialised area, and yet there is little formal education into its intricacies. It is, for most professionals in this area, something they acquired in the course of their daily work. A fuller education structure is necessary, possibly allied to rehabilitation departments in larger centres. Brain injury rehabilitation techniques are powerful tools in the hands of therapy staff and, like effective medical treatments, are capable of misuse. More harm than good can be done by well-meaning, though misconceived, treatment methods; for example, wasting the patient's valuable rehabilitation time through the use of techniques that are outmoded and have been proven ineffective.

This book suggests the adoption of a particular model of brain injury rehabilitation. This is not to say it is perfect or beyond criticism, although because of its nature it is possible to specify goals and to allow for research into the efficacy of treatment.

The need for research into treatment effectiveness has been stated by Gloag (1985b), who suggests that reliable data on the real value of the various interventions are scanty, in spite of many articles proposing ideas and methods. It is also suggested that, even when the treatment is statistically effective, the approach is too time-consuming in relation to the actual functional gains (Miller, 1984). It is necessary to consider the significance of outcome for the patient, rather than the statistical significance required for publication in learned journals. The central consideration must be quality of life for the patient and his or her family.

The problems of families can be various and considerable (Livingston, 1986b), and their needs should be addressed by the treatment team. It is easy to focus attention upon the patient's needs to the exclusion of the needs of the family, especially if members of the family have become useful additions to the treatment team. Organisations such as Headway (in the UK) and the National Head Injury Foundations Inc. (in the USA) provide support for the families of brain-injured patients. They are charitable organisations, lobbying for improved care for the brain-injured patient, and all those involved in brain injury rehabilitation should support this work.

THE ORGANISATION OF PATIENT CARE

The progression and eventual outcome of patients can vary in a number of ways.

Some patients will recover so rapidly that admission to a rehabilitation unit will be unnecessary and the patient will be discharged from the acute-care setting. Appropriate follow-up is necessary to detect problems that may arise later, such as headaches, postural giddiness and poor concentration (Jennett, 1975).

A second group of patients will require the work of a rehabilitation unit but will none the less attain a level of performance equipping them for independent community living.

A further group will, after following a standard rehabilitation programme, retain deficits, the severity of which will seriously compromise their ability to function independently in the community. The patient may progress to a transitional living centre (see below) where the focus will be on training skills, achieving an adjustment to disability and determining what support is required to allow the patient to function at his/her highest level. Their support services may range from day programmes to sheltered work, or possibly receiving supervision of money management and long-term planning.

Another group of patients present such intractable problems that they cannot be managed at the above setting and require a unit specialised in behaviour management.

A final group will have deficits so severe that they require nursing-home care.

Although appropriate management in the acute setting is becoming more common, services are lacking for those with continuing impairments. One facet of a more integrated approach is the transitional living centre (TLC), pioneered in California and established on the model of a therapeutic community (Belanger *et al.*, 1985). Ideally this should be located close to community resources, such as a bank, shops and public transport. This type of setting can provide a transition from institution to community, and can allow patients and their families to accommodate at a psychological and practical level to each patient's relatively fixed cognitive deficits.

A TLC cannot stand independently, however, and needs work and educational programmes to complement its services (Cole *et al.*, 1985).

The needs of the patient and his/her family would be best served by developing a structure of rehabilitation services that give a far greater range of facilities than presently exist (see Figure 11.1). This figure proposes a tentative structure of rehabilitation services. It will be apparent that progression is not necessarily linear from acute setting to the community. Movement throughout the system is flexible, with a variety of units responding to needs at different times. Inherent in this model is the principle that rehabilitation team involvement should not cease when the patient returns to community living.

With the model proposed in this book, brain injury rehabilitation is approaching what for many is the accepted phil-

Figure 11.1: Rehabilitation services structure

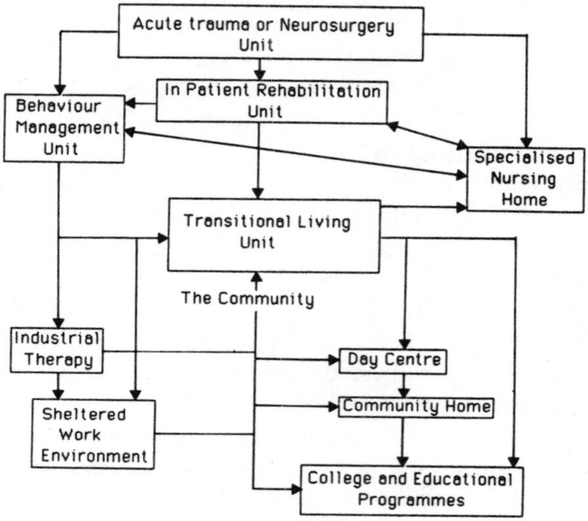

osophy of continuing care of the patient and the family as long as necessary. For many patients this will be the remainder of their lives.

References and Further Reading

Achte, K. A., Hillbom, E. and Aalberg, V. (1969) Psychoses following war brain injuries. *Acta Psychiatrica Scandinavica, 45*, 1–18

Acton, N. (1982) The world's response to disability: evolution of a philosophy. *Archives of Physical Medicine and Rehabilitation, 63*, 145–9

Adams, J. A. (1971) A closed loop theory of motor learning. *Journal of Motor Behaviour 3*, 111–49

Adams, J. A. (1976) A closed loop theory of motor learning. In Stelmach, G. E. (ed.), *Motor control: issues and trends*, Academic Press, London

Adams, J. A. (1977) Feedback theory of how joint receptors regulate the timing and positioning of a limb. *Psychological Review, 84*, 504–23

Alderman, N. (1986) Improving motivational states in the brain injured: preliminary attempts at validating an explanatory model. Unpublished M.App.Sci. thesis, University of Glasgow

Allen, K. E. and Harris, F. R. (1968) Elimination of a child's excessive scratching by training the mother in reinforcement procedures. *Behaviour Research and Therapy, 4*, 78–84

Anderson, D. W. and McLaurin, R. L. (1980) The national head and spinal injury survey. *Journal of Neurosurgery* (supplement), S21

Arts, W. F. M., Van Dongen, H. R., Van Hof-Van Duin, J. and Lamens, E. (1985) Unexpected improvement after prolonged post-traumatic vegetative state. *Journal of Neurology, Neurosurgery and Psychiatry, 48*, 1300–3

Aten, J. L. (1983) Treatment of spastic dysarthria. In Perkins, W. H. (ed.), *Dysarthria and apraxia*, Thième-Stratton, New York

Avorn, J. and Langer, E. (1982) Induced disability in nursing home patients: a controlled trial. *Journal of the American Geriatrics Society, 30*, 397–400

Azrin, N. H. and Foxx, R. M. (1974) *Toilet training in less than a day*, Simon and Schuster, New York

Azrin, N. H. and Nunn, R. G. (1974) A rapid method of eliminating stuttering by a regulated breathing approach. *Behaviour Research and Therapy, 8*, 330

Azrin, N. H. and Wesolowski, M. D. (1974) Theft reversal: an overcorrection procedure for eliminating stealing by retarded persons. *Journal of Applied Behaviour Analysis, 7*, 577–81

Azrin, N. H. and Wesolowski, M. D. (1975) The use of positive practice to eliminate persistent floor sprawling by profoundly retarded persons. *Journal of Applied Behaviour Analysis, 6*, 627–32

Azrin, N. H., Gotlieb, L., Hughort, T. L., Wesolowski, M. D. and Rahn, T. (1975) Eliminating self-injurious behaviour by educative procedures. *Behaviour Research and Therapy, 13*, 101–11

Azrin, N. H., Kaplan, J. and Foxx, R. M. (1973a) Autism reversal:

eliminating stereotyped self-stimulation of retarded individuals. *American Journal of Mental Deficiency, 78*, 241–8

Azrin, N. H., Sneed, T. J. and Foxx, R. M. (1974) Dry-bed training: rapid elimination of childhood enuresis. *Behaviour Research and Therapy, 12*, 147–56

Bach-y-Rita, P. (ed.) (1980) *Recovery of function: theoretical considerations for brain injury rehabilitation*, University Park Press, Baltimore

Bach-y-Rita, P. (1981) Brain plasticity as a basis for the development of rehabilitation procedures for hemiplegia. *Scandinavian Journal of Rehabilitation Medicine, 13*, 73–83

Bach-y-Rita, P. (1983) Introduction: rehabilitation following brain damage: some neurophysiological mechanisms. *International Rehabilitation Medicine, 4*, 165

Bach-y-Rita, P. and Balliet, R. (1986) Recovery from stroke. In Duncan, P. W. and Badke, M. B. (eds), *Motor deficits following stroke*, Year Book Publishers, Chicago

Bach-y-Rita, P., Lazarus, J. C., Boyson, M. G., Balliet, R. and Myers, T. (1987) Neural aspect of motor function as a basis of early and post-acute rehabilitation. In Delisa, J.A., Currie, D., Gans, B., Gatens, P., Leonard, J.A., and McPhee, M. (eds), *Principles and practice of rehabilitation medicine*, J. B. Lippincott, Philadelphia

Bailey, J. and Myerson, L. (1973) Effects of vibratory stimulation on a retardate's self-injurious behaviour. In Ashem, B. and Posner, E. (eds), *Adaptive learning: behaviour modification with children*, Guildford Press, New York

Balliet, R. and Nakayama, K. (1978) Egocentric orientation is influenced by trained voluntary cyclorotory eye movements. *Nature, 257*, 214–15

Bandura, A. A. (1969) *Principles of behavior modification*, Holt, Rinehart and Winston, New York

Barlow, D. H. (1972) Aversive procedures. In Agras, W. S. (ed.), *Behaviour modification: principles and clinical applications*, Churchill/Livingstone, London

Barlow, H. B. (1985) Perception: what quantitative laws govern the acquisition of knowledge from the senses? In Coen, C. W. (ed.), *Functions of the brain*, Clarendon Press, Oxford

Baron, J. C., Bousser, M. G., Comar, D. and Castaigne, P. (1980) 'Crossed cerebellar diaschisis' in human supratentorial brain infarction. *Annals of Neurology, 8*, 128

Bates, P. (1980) The effectiveness of interpersonal skills training on the social skill acquisition of moderately and mildly retarded adults. *Journal of Applied Behaviour Analysis, 12*, 199–210

Bear, D. M. (1983) Behavioural symptoms in temporal lobe epilepsy. *Archives of General Psychiatry, 40*, 467–8

Becker, D. P., Miller, J. D., Ward, J. D., Greenberg, R. P., Young, H. R. and Sakalas, R. (1977) The outcome of severe head injury with early diagnosis and intensive management. *Journal of Neurosurgery, 47*, 491–502

Belanger, S., Berrol, S., Cole, J.R., Fryer, J. and Lock, M. (1985) Bay Area Head Injury Recovery Centre: a therapeutic community. *Cognitive Rehabilitation*, May/June

Bellack, A.S., Hersen, M. and Turner, S.M. (1976) Generalization effects of social skills training in chronic schizophrenics: an experimental analysis. *Behaviour Research and Therapy, 14*, 391–8.

Bennet-Levy, J. and Powell, G. E. (1980) The subjective memory questionnaire (SMQ). An investigation into the reporting of 'real-life' memory skills. *British Journal of Social and Clinical Psychology, 19*, 177–88.

Benson, D. F. (1985) Aphasia. In Heilman, K. M. and Valenstein, E. (eds), *Clinical Neuropsychology*, 2nd edn, Oxford University Press, New York

Berger, M. S., Pitts, L. H., Lovely, M., Edwards, M. S. and Bartowski, H. M. (1985) Outcome from severe head injury in children and adolescents. *Journal of Neurosurgery, 62*, 194–9

Berrol, S. (1986) Evolution and the persistent vegetative state. *Journal of Head Trauma Rehabilitation, 1*, 7–13

Bigler, E. D. and Nangle, R. I. (1985) Case studies in cerebral plasticity. *International Journal of Clinical Neuropsychology, 7*, 12–23

Binder, L. M. (1986) Persisting symptoms after mild head injury: a review of the post-concussive syndrome. *Journal of Clinical and Experimental Neuropsychology, 8*, 323–46

Bird, A. M. and Rikli, R. (1983) Observational learning and practice variability. *Research Quarterly for Exercise and Sport, 54*, 1–4.

Birley, J. and Hudson, B. (1983) The family, the social worker and rehabilitation. In Watts, F. N. and Bennett, D. H. (eds), *Theory and practice of psychiatric rehabilitation*, John Wiley, Chichester

Bizzi, E. and Polit, A. (1979) Processes controlling visually evoked movements. *Neuropsychologica, 17*, 203–13

Bjoneby, E. R. and Reinuang, I. R. (1985) Acquiring and maintaining self-care skills after stroke. *Scandinavian Journal of Rehabilitation Medicine, 17*, 75–80

Blumer, D. (1970) Hypersexual episodes in temporal lobe epilepsy. *American Journal of Psychiatry, 126*, 1099–1106

Bobath, B. (1978) *Adult hemiplegia: evaluation and treatment*, William Heinemann, London

Bolles, R. C. (1979) *Learning Theory*, 2nd edn, Holt, Rinehart and Winston, New York

Bond, M. R. (1975) Assessment of psychosocial outcome after severe head injury. In *Outcome of Severe Damage to the Central Nervous System*. Ciba Foundation Symposium 34, Elsevier, North Holland

Bond, M. R. (1979) The stages of recovery from severe head injury with special reference to late outcome. *International Rehabilitation Medicine, 1*, 155–9

Bornstein, P. H., Bach, P. J., McFall, A. M., Friman, P. C. and Lyons, P. D. (1980) Application of a social skills training programme in the modification of interpersonal skills deficits amongst retarded adults: a clinical replication study. *Journal of Applied Behavior Analysis, 13*, 171–6

Brame, J. M. (1979) The effects of expectancy and previous task cues on motor performance. *Journal of Motor Behaviour, 11*, 215–23

Brandling, R. (1984) *What the papers said*, Edward Arnold, London

Bremer, A. M., Yamada, K. and West, C. R. (1980) Ischemic cerebral oedema in primates: effects of acetazolamide, phenytoin, sorbitol, dexamethasone, and methylprednisolone on brain water and electrolytes. *Neurosurgery, 6* (2), 149–54

Brinkman, R., Von Cramon, D. and Schultz, H. (1976) Munich Coma Scale (MCS). *Journal of Neurology, Neurosurgery and Psychiatry, 39*, 788–93

Brocklehurst, J. C., Andrews, K., Richards, B. and Laycock, P. J. (1978) How much physical therapy for patients with stroke? *British Medical Journal, 1*, 307–10

Broen, L., Branston-McClean, M., Baumgart, D., Vincent, L., Falvey, M. and Schroeder, J. (1979) Using the characteristics of current and subsequent least restrictive environments in the development of content for severely handicapped students. *AAESPH Review, 4*, 407–24

Brooks, D. N. (1984) *Closed head injury: psychological, social and family consequences*, Oxford University Press, Oxford

Brooks, D. N. and McKinlay, W. (1983) Personality and behavioural change after severe blunt head injury — a relative's view. *Journal of Neurology, Neurosurgery and Psychiatry, 46*, 336–44

Brooks, D. N., Campsie, L., Symington, C., Beattie, A. and McKinlay, W. (1986) The five year outcome of severe blunt head injury: a relative's view. *Journal of Neurology, Neurosurgery and Psychiatry, 49*, 764–70

Bucher, B. and Lovaas, O. I. (1967) Use of aversive stimulation in behaviour modification. In Jones, M. R. (ed.), *Miami Symposium on the Prediction of Behaviour, 1967: aversive stimulation*, University of Miami Press, Coral Gables, Florida

Burgess, P., Mitchelmore, S. and Giles, G. M. (1987) Operational aspects of attention in atypical mental impairment: a behavioural treatment procedure. *American Journal of Occupational Therapy* (in press)

Calculator, S. and Luchko, C. (1983) Evaluating the effectiveness of a communication board training program. *Journal of Speech and Hearing Disorders, 48*, 185–91

Cannon, W. B. and Rosenblueth, A. (1949) *The supersensitivity of denervated structures*, Macmillan, New York

Capaldi, E. J. (1967) A sequential hypothesis of instrumental learning. In Spence, K. W. and Spence, J. T. (eds), *The psychology of learning and motivation*, vol. 1, Academic Press, New York

Carson, L. M. and Wiegand, R. L. (1979) Motor schema formation and retention in young children: a test of Schmidt's schema theory. *Journal of Motor Behaviour, 11*, 247–51

Cartlidge, N. E. F. (1978) Post-concussional syndrome. *Scottish Medical Journal, 23*, 103

Casson, I. R., Sham. R., Campebell, E. A., Tarlau, M. and Didomenico, A. (1982) Neurologic and CT evaluation of knocked-out boxers. *Journal of Neurology, Neurosurgery and Psychiatry, 45*, 170–4

Catalano, J. F. and Kleiner, B. M. (1984) Distant transfer in coincident timing as a function of variability in practice. *Perceptual and Motor Skills, 58*, 851–6

Cermak, L. S. (1976) The encoding capacity of a patient with amnesia due to encephalitis. *Neuropsychologia, 14*, 311–26

Cohen, R. E. (1986) Behavioral treatment of incontinence in a profoundly neurologically impaired adult. *Archives of Physical Medicine and Rehabilitation, 67*, 833–84

Cohen, S. B. (1986) Educational reintegration and programming for children with head injuries. *Journal of Head Trauma Rehabilitation, 1*, 22–9

Cohen, S. B., Joyce, C. M., Rhoades, K. W. and Welks, D. M. (1985) Educational programming for head-injured students. In Ylvisaker, M. (ed.), *Head injury rehabilitation: children and adolescents.* College-Hill Press, San Diego

Cole, J. R., Cope, N. and Cervelli, L. (1985) Rehabilitation of the severely brain injured patient: a community-based, low-cost model program. *Archives of Physical Medicine and Rehabilitation, 66*, 38–40

Coleman, C. L., Cook, A. M. and Myer, L. S. (1980) Assessing non-oral clients for assistive communication devices. *Journal of Speech and Hearing Disorders, 45*, 515–26

Colohan, A. R. T., Dacey, R. G., Alves, W. M., Rimel, R. W. and Jane, J. A. (1986) Neurologic and neurosurgical implications of mild head injury. *Journal of Head Trauma Rehabilitation, 1*, 13–21

Cope, D. N. (1985) Traumatic closed head injury; status of rehabilitation treatment. *Seminars in Neurology, 5*, 212–20

Cope, D. N. and Hall, K. (1982) Head injury rehabilitation: benefits of early intervention. *Archives of Physical Medicine and Rehabilitation, 63*, 433–7

Cottam, P. and Sutton, A. (1985) *Conductive education: a system for overcoming motor disorder.* Croom Helm, London

Cotton, E. (1965) The Institute for Movement Therapy and School for Conductors, Budapest, Hungary. *Developmental Medicine and Child Neurology, 7*, 437–46

Cotton, E. and Kinsman, R. (1983) *Conductive education for adult hemiplegia,* Churchill Livingstone, London

Craighead, W. E., Kazdin, A. E. and Mahoney, M. J. (1976) *Behaviour modification: principles, issues and applications,* Houghton Mifflin, Boston

Craik, F. I. M. and Lockhart, R. S. (1972) Levels of processing: a framework for memory research. *Journal of Verbal Learning and Verbal Behaviour, 11*, 671–84

Crosson, B. and Buenning, W. (1984) An individualized memory retraining program after closed head-injury: a single case study. *Journal of Clinical Neuropsychology, 6*, 287–301

Culshaw, C. and Waters, D. (1976) *Headwork, Books 1–4*, Oxford University Press, Oxford

Cummings, J. L., Benson, D. F., Walsh, M. J. and Levine, H. L. (1979) Left to right transfer of language dominance: a case study. *Neurology, 29*, 1547–50

Cuvo, A. J. and Davis, P. K. (1983) Behaviour therapy and community living skills. In Hersen, M., Eisler, R. M. and Miller, P.M. (eds), *Progress in behaviour modification*, vol. 14, Academic Press, New York

Damasio, A. R. (1985) The frontal lobes. In Heilman, K. M. and Valenstein, E. (eds), *Clinical neuropsychology*, 2nd edn, Oxford University Press, New York

Darley, F. L., Aronson, A. E. and Brown, J. R. (1975) *Motor speech disorders*, Saunders, Philadelphia

Davey, G. (1981) Conditioning principles, behaviourism and behaviour therapy. In Davey, G. (ed.), *Applications of conditioning theory*, Methuen, London

Davidoff, G., Morris, J., Roth, E. and Bleiberg, J. (1985a) Closed head injury in spinal cord injured patients: Retrospective study of loss of consciousness and post traumatic amnesia. *Archives of Physical Medicine and Rehabilitation, 66*, 41–3

Davidoff, G., Morris, J., Roth, E. and Bleiberg, J. (1985b) Cognitive dysfunction and mild closed head injury in traumatic spinal cord injury. *Archives of Physical Medicine and Rehabilitation, 66*, 489–91

Deal, J. L. and Florance, C. I. (1978) Modification of the 8 step continuum for the treatment of apraxia of speech in adults. *Journal of Speech and Hearing Disorders, 43*, 89–95

Deitz, S. M. (1977) An analysis of programming schedules in educational settings. *Behaviour Research and Therapy, 15*, 103–11

Denker, P. G. (1944) Postconcussion syndrome: prognosis and evaluation of organic factors. *New York State Journal of Medicine, 44*, 379–84

Devor, M. (1982) Plasticity in the adult nervous system. In Illis, L. S., Sedgwick, E. M. and Glanville, H. J. (eds), *Rehabilitation of the neurological patient*, Blackwell Scientific Publications, Oxford

Dikman, S., McClean, A. and Temkin, N. (1986) Neuropsychological and psychosocial consequences of minor head injury. *Journal of Neurology, Neurosurgery and Psychiatry, 49*, 1227–32

Diller, L., Ben-Yishay, Y., Gerstman, L. J., Goodkin, R., Gordon, W. and Weinberg, J. (1974) Studies in cognitive rehabilitation in hemiplegia. *Rehabilitation Monograph No. 50*, Institute of Rehabilitation Medicine, New York University Medical Center

Dolan, M. P. (1979) The use of contingent reinforcement for improving the personal appearance and hygiene of chronic psychiatric inpatients. *Journal of Clinical Psychology, 35*, 140–4

Dolan, M. P. and Norton, J. C. (1977) A programmed training technique that uses reinforcement to facilitate acquisition and retention in brain damaged patients. *Journal of Clinical Psychology, 33*, 496–501

Eames, P. and Wood, R. Ll. (1985a) Rehabilitation after severe brain injury: a follow-up study of a behaviour modification approach. *Journal of Neurology, Neurosurgery and Psychiatry, 48*, 613–19

Eames, P. and Wood, R. Ll. (1985b) Rehabilitation after severe brain injury: a special-unit approach to behaviour disorders. *International Rehabilitation Medicine, 7*, 130–3

Edelstein, B. and Eisler, R. M. (1976) Effects of modeling and modeling with instructions and feedback on the behavioural components of social skills with schizophrenics. *Behaviour Therapy, 7*, 382–9

Elisinger, P. and Damasio, A. R. (1984) Behavioural disturbances associated with rupture of anterior communicating artery aneurysms. *Seminars in Neurology, 4*, 385–9

Ellis, N. (1970) Memory processes in retardates and normals. *International Review of Research in Mental Retardation, 4*, 1–31

Emerick, L. L. and Hatton, J. T. (1974) *Diagnosis and evaluation in speech pathology*, Prentice-Hall, Englewood Cliffs, New Jersey

Evans, C. D., Bull, C. P. I., Devonport, M. J., Hall, P. M., Jones, J., Middleton, F. R. I., Russell, G., Stichbury, J. C. and Whitehead, B. (1981) Rehabilitation of the brain-damaged survivor. *Injury, 8*, 80–97

Feigenson, J. S., McCarthay, M. L., Meese, P. D. and Feigenson, W. D. (1977) Stroke rehabilitation, factors predicting outcome and length of stay: an overview. *New York State Journal of Medicine, 9*, 1426–30

Finger, S. and Stein, D. G. (1982) *Brain damage and recovery*, Academic Press, New York

Fitts, P. M. (1964) Perceptual-motor skill learning. In Melton, A. M. (ed.), *Categories of human learning*, Academic Press, New York

Fitts, P. M. and Posner, M. I. (1967) *Human performance*, Brooks/Cole, Belmont, California

Fordyce, D. J., Roueche, J. R. and Prigatano, G. P. (1985) Enhanced emotional reactions in chronic head trauma patients. *Journal of Neurology, Neurosurgery and Psychiatry, 48*, 876–81

Foxx, R. M. and Azrin, N. H. (1972) Restitution: a method of eliminating aggressive disruptive behaviour of retarded and brain damaged patients. *Behaviour Research and Therapy, 10*, 15–27

Foxx, R. M. and Azrin, N. H. (1973) Dry pants: a rapid method of toilet training children. *Behaviour Research and Therapy, 11*, 435–42

Foxx, R. M. and Martin, E. D. (1975) Treatment of scavenging behaviour by overcorrection. *Behaviour Research and Therapy, 13*, 153–62

Freed, W. J., Medinaceli, L. and Wyatt, R. J. (1985) Promoting functional plasticity in the damaged nervous system. *Science, 227*, 1544–52

Friedman, R. B. and Alpert, M.L. (1985) Alexia. In Heilman, K. M. and Valenstein, E. (eds), *Clinical neuropsychology*, 2nd edn, Oxford University Press, New York

Fukuyama, H., Kameyama, M., Harada, K. (1986) Thalamic tumours invading the brain stem produce crossed cerebellar diaschisis demonstrated by PET. *Journal of Neurology, Neurosurgery, and Psychiatry, 49*, 524–8

Fussey, I. and Tyerman, D. (1985) An exploration of memory retraining following closed head injury. *International Journal of Rehabilitation Research, 8*, 465–7

Gazzaniga, M. S. (1978) Is seeing believing: notes on clinical recovery. In Finger, S. (ed.), *Recovery from brain damage: research and theory*, Plenum Press, New York

Gennarelli, T. A., Spielman, G. M., Langfitt, T. W., Gildenberg, P. L., Harrington, T., Jane, J. A., Marshall, L. F., Miller, J. D. and Pitts, L. H. (1982) Influence of the type of intracranial lesion on outcome from severe head injury. *Journal of Neurosurgery, 56*, 26–32

Gent, A. and Giles, G. M. (1986) A clever combination — the key to treating the brain-injured. *Therapy*, 22 January

Gianutsos, R. (1980) What is cognitive rehabilitation? *Journal of Rehabilitation, 46*, 36–40

Gianutsos, R. (1981) Training the short- and long-term verbal recall of a post-encephalitic amnesic. *Journal of Clinical Neuropsychology, 3*, 143–53

Gianutsos, R. and Grynbaum, B. B. (1983) Helping brain-injured people to contend with hidden cognitive deficits. *International Rehabilitation Medicine, 5*, 37–40

Gibson, J. J. (1950) *The perception of the visual world*, Houghton-Mifflin, Boston

Gibson, J. J. (1966) *The senses considered as perceptual systems*, Houghton-Mifflin, Boston

Gibson, J. J. (1979) *The ecological approach to visual perception*, Houghton-Mifflin, Boston

Gilchrist, E. and Wilkinson, M. (1979) Some factors determining prognosis in young people with severe head injury. *Archives of Neurology, 36*, 355–9

Glasgow, R. E., Zeiss, R. A., Barrera, M. and Lewinsohn, P. M. (1977) Case studies on remediating memory deficits in brain damaged individuals. *Journal of Clinical Psychology, 33*, 1049–54

Glass, A. V., Gazzaniga, M. S. and Premack, D. (1973) Artificial language training in global aphasias. *Neuropsychologia, 2*, 95–103

Glick, S. D. and Greenstein, S. (1973) Possible modulatory influences of frontal cortex on nigro-striatal function. *British Journal of Pharmacology, 49*, 316–21

Glisky, E. L., Schacter, D. L. and Tulving, E. (1986) Computer learning by memory-impaired patients: acquisition and retention of complex knowledge. *Neuropsychologia, 24*, 313–28

Gloag, D. (1985b) Rehabilitation after head injury: 2. behaviour and emotional problems, long term needs, and the requirements for services. *British Medical Journal, 290*, 913–16

Gloag, D. (1985a) Services for people with head injuries. *British Medical Journal, 291*, 557–8

Goldenson, R. M., Dunham, J. R. and Dunham, C. F. (1978)

Disability and rehabilitation handbook, McGraw-Hill, New York

Goldstein, G. and Ruthven, L. (1983) *Rehabilitation of the brain damaged adult,* Plenum Press, New York

Goldstein, G., Ryan, C., Turner, S. M., Kanagy, M., Barry, K. and Kelly, L. (1985) Three methods of memory training for severely amnesic patients. *Behaviour Modification, 9*(9), 357–74

Goldstein, L. H. and Oakley, D. A. (1985) Expected and actual behavioural capacity after diffuse reduction in cerebral cortex: a review and suggestions for rehabilitative techniques with the mentally handicapped and head injured. *British Journal of Clinical Psychology, 24,* 13–24

Goodglass, H. and Kaplan, E. (1972) *The assessment of aphasia and related disorders,* Lea and Febiger, Philadelphia

Goodkin, R. (1966) Case studies in behavioural research and rehabilitation. *Perceptual and Motor Skills, 23,* 171–82

Goodkin, R. (1969) Changes in word modification, sentence production and relevance in an aphasic through verbal conditioning. *Behaviour Research and Therapy, 7,* 93

Goodman-Smith, A. and Turnbull, J. (1983) A behavioural approach to the rehabilitation of severely brain injured adults: an illustrated case history. *Physiotherapy, 69,* 393–6

Gordon, W. A., Hibbard, M. R., Egelko, S., Diller, L., Shaver, M. S., Lieberman, A. and Ragnarsson, K. (1985) Perceptual remediation in patients with right brain damage: a comprehensive program. *Archives of Physical Medicine and Rehabilitation, 66,* 353–9

Grafman, J. (1983) Memory assessment and remediation in brain injured patients: from theory to practice. In Edelstein, B. A. and Couture, E. T. (eds), *Behavioural assessment and rehabilitation of the traumatically brain damaged,* Plenum Press, New York

Gronwall, D. and Wrightson, P. (1975) Cumulative effects of concussion. *Lancet, ii,* 995–7

Hall, K., Cope, N. and Rappaport, M. (1985) Glasgow outcome scale and disability rating scale: comparative usefulness in following recovery in traumatic head injury. *Archives of Physical Rehabilitation and Medicine, 66,* 35–7

Harris, J. (1984) Methods of improving memory. In Wilson, B. and Moffat, M. (eds), *Clinical management of memory disorders,* Croom Helm, London

Hartman, J. (1987) Alteration in patterns of urinary elimination. In Carpenito, L. J. (ed.), *Nursing diagnosis,* J. B. Lippincott, Philadelphia

Hawkins, C. A., Mellanby, J. and Brown, J. (1985) Antiepileptic and antiamnesic effect of carbamazepine in experimental limbic epilepsy. *Journal of Neurology, Neurosurgery and Psychiatry, 48,* 459–68

Hawley, L. A. (1984) *A family guide to the rehabilitation of the severely head injured patient,* Healthcare International, Austin, Texas

Hecaen, H. and Albert, M. L. (1978) *Human neuropsychology,* Wiley, New York

Heiskanen, O. and Kaste, M. (1974) Late prognosis of severe brain injury in children. *Developmental Medicine and Child Neurology, 16*, 11–14

Ho, L. and Shea, J. B. (1979) Orienting task specificity in incidental motor learning. *Journal of Motor Behaviour, 11*, 135–40

Holland, A. L. (1980) *Communicative abilities in daily living.* University Park Press, Baltimore

Holland, L. K. and Whalley, M. J. (1981) The work of a psychiatrist in a rehabilitation hospital. *British Journal of Psychiatry, 138*, 222–9

Holt, K. S. (1975) A single nurse–teacher–therapist. *Child Care, Health and Development, 1*. 45–50

Horton, A. M. and Howe, N. R. (1981) Behavioural treatment of the traumatically brain injured: a case study. *Perceptual and Motor Skills, 53*, 349–50

Horton, A. M. and Miller, W. G. (1985) Neuropsychology and behaviour therapy. In Hersen, M., Eisler, R. M. and Miller, P. M. (eds), *Progress in behaviour modification*, vol. 19, Academic Press, Orlando

Hoshmand, H. and Brawley, B. W. (1970) Temporal lobe seizures and exhibitionism. *Neurology, 9*, 1119–24

Hull, C. L. (1943) *Principles of behaviour*, Appleton-Century-Crofts, New York

Hull, C. L. (1952) *A behaviour system: an introduction to behaviour theory concerning the individual organism*, Yale University Press, New Haven

Husak, W. S. and Reeve, T. G. (1979) Novel response production as a function of variability and amount of practice. *Research Quarterly, 50*, 215–21

Illis, L. S. (1983) Determinants of recovery. *International Rehabilitation Medicine, 4*, 166–72

Ince, L. P. (1973) Behavior modification with an aphasic man. *Rehabilitation Research Practice Review, 4*, 37

Iwata, B. A., Dorsey, M. F., Slifer, K. J., Bauman, K. E. and Richman, C. S. Towards a functional analysis of self-injury. *Analysis and Intervention in Developmental Disabilities, 2*, 3–20

Jellinek, H. M. and Harvey, R. F. (1982) Vocational/educational services in a medical rehabilitation facility: outcomes in spinal cord and brain injured patients. *Archives of Physical Medicine and Rehabilitation, 63*, 87–8

Jennett, B. (1975) Who cares for head injuries? *British Medical Journal, 3*, 267–70

Jennett, B. (1982) Chairman of Co-ordinating Group. Research aspects of rehabilitation after brain injury in adults. *Lancet, ii*, 1034–6

Jennett, B. and Bond, M. R. (1975) Assessment of outcome after severe brain injury. *Lancet, i*, 480–4

Jennett, B. and Plum, F. (1979) Persistent vegetative state after brain damage. A syndrome in search of a name. *Lancet, i*, 734–7

Jennett, B. and Teasdale, G. (1981) *Management of head injuries*, F. A. Davis, Philadelphia

Jennett, B., Snoek, J., Bond, R. and Brooks, D. N. (1981) Disability after severe head injury: observations on the Glasgow Outcome Scale. *Journal of Neurology, Neurosurgery and Psychiatry, 44*, 285–93

Jennett, B., and Teasdale, G. and Galbraith, S. (1977) Severe head injuries in three countries. *Journal of Neurology, Neurosurgery and Psychiatry, 40*, 291–8

Jennett, B., Teather, D. and Bennie, S. (1973) Epilepsy after head injury. *Lancet, 305*, 652–3

Jennett, W. B. (1962) *Epilepsy after blunt head injuries*, Heinemann, London

Johnson, R. and McCabe, J. (1982) Schema theory: a test of the hypothesis, variation in practice. *Perceptual and Motor Skills, 55*, 231–4

Johnson, W., Darley, F. L. and Darley, D. C. (1963) *Diagnostic methods in speech pathology*, Harper and Row, New York

Kazdin, A. E. and Bootzin, R. R. (1972) The token economy: an evaluative review. *Journal of Applied Behaviour Analysis, 5*, 343–72

Kertesz, A. (1982) *The Western Aphasia battery*, Grune and Stratton, New York

Kertesz, A. (1985) Recovery and treatment. In Heilman, K. M. and Valenstein, E. (eds), *Clinical neuropsychology*, Oxford University Press, New York

Kertesz, A. and Poole, E. (1974) The aphasia quotient: the taxonomic approach to measurement of aphasic disability. *Canadian Journal of Neurological Science*, 1, 7–16

Klauber, M. R., Marshall, L. F., Toole, B. M., Knowleton, S. L. and Bowers, S. A. (1985) Cause of decline in head-injury mortality rate in San Diego County, California. *Journal of Neurosurgery, 62*, 528–31

Klonoff, P. S., Costa, L. D. and Snow, W. G. (1986) Predictors and indicators of quality of life in patients with closed head injury. *Journal of Clinical and Experimental Neuropsychology, 8(5)*, 469–85

Kottke, F. (1982) The neurophysiology of motor function. In Kottke, F., Stillwell, G. K. and Lehmann, J. F. (eds), *Krusen's handbook of physical medicine and rehabilitation*. W. B. Saunders, Philadelphia

Lancet (1982) Research aspects of rehabilitation after acute brain damage in adults. Report of a coordinating group, 6 November, *Lancet, 6*, 1034–6

Lancet (1983) Caring for the disabled after head injury. Editorial, *Lancet, ii*, 948–9

Landis, T., Graves, R., Benson, D. F. and Hebben, N. (1982) Visual recognition through kinaesthetic mediation. *Psychological Medicine, 12*, 515–31

LaPointe, L. L. (1978) Aphasia therapy: some principles and strategies for treatment. In Johns, D. F. (ed.), *Clinical management of neurogenic communicative disorders*, Little, Brown, Boston

Lashley, B. and Drabman, R. (1974) Facilitation of the acquisition and retention of sight–word vocabulary through token reinforcement. *Journal of Applied Behaviour Analysis, 7*, 307–12

Lashley, K. S. (1917) The accuracy of movement in the absence of excitation from the moving organ. *American Journal of Physiology, 43*, 169–94

Laurence, S. and Stein, D. G. (1978) Recovery after brain damage and the concept of localization of function. In Finger, S. (ed.), *Recovery from brain damage*, Plenum Press, New York

Lee, T. D., Magill, R. A. and Weeks, D. J. (1985) Influence of practice schedules on testing schema theory predictions in adults. *Journal of Motor Behavior, 17*, 283–99

Levin, H. S. and Spiers, P. A. (1985) Acalculia. In Heilman, K. M. and Valenstein, E. (eds), *Clinical neuropsychology*, 2nd edn, Oxford University Press, New York

Levin, H. S., Grossman, R. G., Rose, J. E. and Teasdale, M. B. (1979) Long-term neuropsychological outcome of closed head injury. *Journal of Neurosurgery, 50*, 412–22

Lewin, W., Marshall, T. F. De C. and Roberts, A. H. (1979) Long term outcome after severe head injury. *British Medical Journal, 2*, 1533–8

Lezak, M. D. (1976) *Neuropsychological assessment*, Oxford University Press, New York

Lezak, M. D. (1978) Living with the characterologically altered brain-injured patient. *Journal of Clinical Psychiatry, 39*, 592–8

Lincoln, N. B., Whiting, S. E., Cockburn, J. and Bhavnani, G. (1985) An evaluation of perceptual training. *International Rehabilitation Medicine, 7*, 99–110

Lind, K. (1982) A synthesis of studies on stroke rehabilitation. *Journal of Chronic Diseases, 35*, 133–49

Lishman, J. and Lee, D. (1973) The autonomy of visual kinesthesis. *Perception, 2*, 287–94

Lishman, W. A. (1978) *Organic psychiatry*, Blackwell Scientific Publications, Oxford

Liu, C. N. and Chambers, W. W. (1958) Intraspinal sprouting of dorsal root axons. *Archives of Neurology and Psychiatry, 79*, 46–61

Livingston, M. G. (1986a) Assessment of need for coordinated approach in families with victims of head injury. *British Medical Journal, 293*, 742–4

Livingston, M. G. (1986b) Head injury: the relative's response. *Brain Injury, 1*, 8–14

Livingston, M. G. and Livingston, H. M. (1985) The Glasgow assessment schedule: clinical and research assessment of head injury outcome. *International Rehabilitation Medicine, 7*, 145–9

Locke, E. A., Cartledge, N. and Koeppel, J. (1968) Motivational effects of knowledge and results: a goal-setting phenomenon. *Psychological Bulletin, 70*, 458–74

Logigan, M. K., Samuels, M. A., Falconer, J. and Zagar, R. (1983) Clinical exercise trials for stroke patients. *Archives of Physical Medicine and Rehabilitation, 64*, 364–7

London, P. (1972) The end of ideology in behaviour modification. *Annals of Psychology*, 27, 913–20

Long, C. J., Gouvier, W. D. and Cole, J. C. (1984) A model of recovery for the total rehabilitation of the individual with head trauma. *Journal of Rehabilitation*, 50, 39–45

Lord, J. P. and Hall, K. H. (1986) Neuromuscular reeducation versus traditional programs for stroke rehabilitation. *Archives of Physical Medicine and Rehabilitation*, 67, 88–91

Lundgren, C. C. and Persechino, E. L. (1986) Cognitive group: a treatment program for head-injured adults. *American Journal of Occupational Therapy*, 40, 397–401

Luria, A. R. (1961) *The role of speech in the regulation of normal and abnormal behaviour*. Pergamon Press, Oxford

Luria, A. R. (1972) *The man with a shattered world*, Penguin Books, Harmondsworth

Luria, A. R. (1973) *The working brain*, Basic Books, New York

Mackintosh, N. J. (1974) *The psychology of animal learning*, Academic Press, London

Mackintosh, N. J. (1983) *Conditioning and associative learning*, Oxford University Press, Oxford

McFarlain, R. A., Andy, O. J., Scott, R. W. and Wheatley, M. L. (1975) Suppression of head-banging on the ward. *Psychological Reports*, 36, 315–21

McKinlay, W. W., Brooks, D. N. and Bond, M. R. (1983) Post-concussional symptoms, financial compensation and outcome of severe blunt head injury. *Journal of Neurology, Neurosurgery and Psychiatry*, 46, 1084–91

McLaughlin, A. M. and Schaffer, V. (1985) Rehabilitation or remould? Family involvement in head trauma recovery. *Cognitive Rehabilitation*, Jan/Feb.

McQueen, J. K., Blackwood, D. H. R., Harris, P., Kalbag, R. M. and Johnson, A. L. (1983) Low risk of late post-traumatic seizures following severe head injury: implications for clinical trials of prophylaxis. *Journal of Neurology, Neurosurgery and Psychiatry*, 46, 899–904

Measel, C. J. and Alfieri, P. A. (1978) Treatment of self-injurious behaviour by a combination of positive reinforcement for incompatible behaviour and overcorrection. *American Journal of Mental Deficiency*, 81, 147–53

Merksey, H. and Woodforde, J. M. (1972) Psychiatric sequelae of minor head injury. *Brain*, 95, 521–8

Merton, P. A. (1972) How do we control the contraction of our muscles? *Scientific American*, 226, 30–7

Miller, B. L., Cummings, J. L., McIntyre, H., Ebers, G. and Grode, M. (1986) Hypersexuality or altered sexual preference following brain injury. *Journal of Neurology, Neurosurgery and Psychiatry*, 48, 867–73

Miller, E. (1980) The training characteristics of severely head injured patients: a preliminary study. *Journal of Neurology, Neurosurgery and Psychiatry*, 43, 525–8

Miller, E. (1984) *Recovery and management of neuropsychological impairments*, John Wiley, Chichester

Miller, E. (1985) Cognitive retraining of neurological patients. In Watts, F. N. (ed.), *New developments in clinical psychology*, John Wiley, Chichester

Miller, H. (1961) Accident neurosis. *British Medical Journal, i.* 919–25, 992–8

Miller, H. (1966) Mental after-effects of head injury. *Proceedings of the Royal Society of Medicine, 59*, 257–61

Milner, B. (1974) Hemispheric specialization: scope and limits. In Schimitt, F. O. and Worden, F. G. (eds), *The neurosciences: third study program*, MIT Press, Cambridge, Massachusetts

Milton, S. (1985) Compensatory memory strategy training: a practical approach for managing persisting memory problems. *Cognitive Rehabilitation, 3*, 8–16

Moffatt, N. (1984) Strategies of memory therapy. In Wilson, B. and Moffatt, N. (eds), *Clinical management of memory problems*, Aspen Systems Corporation, Tunbridge Wells

Monakow, C. Von (1914) *Das Grosshirn und die Abbavfunktion durch Kortikale*, Bergmann, Herde Weisbaden

Mulder, T. and Hulstijn, W. (1984) The effects of fatigue and task repetition on the surface electromyographic signal. *Psychophysiology, 21*, 528–34

Murphy, G. (1980) Decreasing undesirable behaviours. In Yule, W. and Carr, J. (eds), *Behaviour modification for the mentally handicapped*, Croom Helm, London

Nasher, L. M. and McCollum, G. (1985) The organization of human postural movements: a formal basis and experimental synthesis. *Behavioural and Brain Sciences, 8*, 135–72

Newell, A. and Rosenbloom, P. S. (1981) Mechanisms of skill acquisition and the law of practice. In J. R. Anderson (ed.), *Cognitive skills and their acquisition*, Lawrence Erlbaum Associates.

Novak, T. A., Satterfield, W. T., Lyons, K., Kolski, G., Hackmeyer, L. and Conner, M. (1984) Stroke onset and rehabilitation: time lag as a factor in treatment outcome. *Archives of Physical Medicine and Rehabilitation, 65*, 316–19

Oakley, D. A. (1983) Learning capacity outside the neocortex in animals and man: implications for therapy after brain injury. In Davey, G. (ed.), *Animal models of human behaviour: conceptual, evolutionary and neurobiological perspectives*, Wiley, Chichester

Oddy, M., Humphey, M. and Uttley, D. (1978) Stresses upon the relatives of head-injured patients. *British Journal of Psychiatry, 133*, 507–13

Pantano, J. C., Baron, J. C., Samson, Y., Bousser, M. G., Derouesne, C. and Comar, D. (1968) Crossed cerebellar diachisis: further studies. *Brain, 109*, 677–94

Panting, A. and Merry, P. H. (1972) The long-term rehabilitation of severe head injuries with particular reference to the need for social and medical support for the patient's family. *Rehabilitation, 38,* 33–7

Parasuraman, R. (1984) The psychobiology of sustained attention. In Warm, J. S. (ed.), *Sustained attention in human performance,* John Wiley, Chichester

Patten, B. M. (1972) The ancient art of memory: usefulness in treatment. *Archives of Neurology, 26,* 25–31

Pavlov, I. P. (1927) *Conditioned reflexes,* Oxford University Press, London

Perkins, W. H. (1983) *Dysarthria and apraxia,* Thième-Stratton, New York

Petrides, M. (1985) Deficits on conditional associative-learning tasks after frontal and temporal-lobe lesions in man. *Neuropsychologia, 23,* 601–14

Plum, F. and Posner, J. (1980) *The diagnosis of stupor and coma,* 3rd edn, F. A. Davis, Philadelphia

Posner, M. I. (1975) The psychobiology of attention. In Gazzaniga, M. S. and Blakemore, C. (eds), *Handbook of psychobiology,* Academic Press, New York

Powell, G. E. (1979) *Brain and personality,* Saxon House, Farnborough, Hants

Powell, G. E. (1981) *Brain function therapy,* Gower, Aldershot, Hants

Pribram, K. H. (1968) Towards a neuropsychological theory of person. In Pribram, K. H. (ed.), *The study of personality: an interdisciplinary approach,* Holt, Rinehart and Winston, New York

Prigatano, G. P., Fordyce, D. J., Zeiner, H. K., Roueche, J. R., Pepping, M. and Wood, B. C. (1984) Neuropsychological rehabilitation after closed head injury in young adults. *Journal of Neurology, Neurosurgery and Psychiatry, 47,* 505–13

Rappaport, M., Hall, K. M., Hopkins, K., Belleza, T. and Cope, D. N. (1982) Disability rating scale for severe head trauma: coma to community. *Archives of Physical Medicine and Rehabilitation, 63,* 118–23

Rappaport, M. D., Sonis, W. A., Fialkov, M. J., Matson, J. L. and Kazdin, A. E. (1983) Carbemazepine and behavior therapy. *Behavior Modification, 7,* 255–65

Reason, J. (1979) Action not as planned. In Underwood, G. and Stevens, R. (eds), *Aspects of consciousness, Vol. 1: psychological issues,* Academic Press, London

Reed, E. S. (1982) An outline of a theory of action systems. *Journal of Motor Behaviour, 14,* 98–134

Rey, A. (1959) Le test de copie de figure complex. *Editions Centre de Psychologie Appliqué,* Paris

Ridgeway, W. (1985) *Maths about town,* Edward Arnold, London

Rimel, R. W., Giordani, B., Barth, J. T., Boll, T. J. and Jane, J. A. (1981) Disability caused by minor head injury. *Neurosurgery, 9,* 221–8

Robinson, R. G. and Szetela, B. (1981) Mood change following left hemispheric brain injury. *Annals of Neurology, 9,* 447–53

Robinson, R. O. (1986) Mechanisms of brain recovery. *Journal of the Royal Society of Medicine, 79*, 430–3

Rose, M. (1980) Rehabilitation after head injury. In Nichols, P. J. R. (ed.), *Rehabilitation medicine*, Butterworths, London

Rosenbeck, J. C., Lemme, M. L., Ahern, M. B., Harris, E. H. and Wertz, R. T. (1973) A treatment for apraxia of speech in adults. *Journal of Speech and Hearing Disorders, 38*, 462–72

Rothi, L. J. and Horner, J. (1983) Restitution and substitution: two theories of recovery with application to neurobehavioural treatment. *Journal of Clinical Neuropsychology, 5*, 73–81

Rusk, H. A., Block, J. M. and Lowman, E. W. (1969) Rehabilitation following severe brain damage: immediate and long term follow-up results in 27 cases. *Medical Clinics of North America, 53*, 677–84

Russell, W. R. and Smith, A. (1961) Post-traumatic amnesia in closed head injuries. *Archives of Neurology, 5*, 16–29

Sabel, B. A. and Stein, D. G. (1986) Pharmacological treatment of central nervous system injury. *Nature, 323*, 493

Salmoni, A. W., Schmidt, R. A. and Walter, C. B. (1984) Knowledge of results and motor learning: A review and critical reappraisal. *Psychological Bulletin, 95*, 355–86

Sarno, M. T. (1984) Verbal impairment after closed head injury. Report of a replication study. *Journal of Nervous and Mental Diseases, 172*, 475–9

Schmidt, B. (1969) Occupational rehabilitation of the brain injured worker. In Walker, A. E., Caveness, W. F. and Critchley, M. (eds), *The late effects of head injury*, Thomas, Springfield, Illinois

Schmidt, R. A. (1975) A schema theory of discrete motor skill learning. *Psychological Review, 82*, 225–60

Schmidt, R. A. (1976) The schema as a solution to the persistent problems in motor learning theory. In Stelmach, G. E. (ed.), *Motor control: issues and trends*, Academic Press, London

Schmidt, R. A. (1980) On the theoretical status of time in motor program representations. In Stelmach, G. E. and Requin, J. (eds), *Tutorials in motor behavior*, North Holland, Amsterdam

Schmidt, R. A. (1982) More on motor programs. In Kelso, J. A. S. (ed.), *Human motor behaviour: an introduction*, Laurence Erlbaum, New Jersey

Schneider, W., Dumais, S. T. and Shiffrin, R. M. (1984) Automatic and controlled processing and attention. In Parasuraman, R. and Davis, D. R. (eds), *Varieties of attention*, Academic Press, London

Schoenfeld, T. A. and Hamilton, L. W. (1977) Secondary brain changes following lesions: a new paradigm for lesion experimentation. *Physiology and Behavior, 18*, 951–67

Schuell, H. (1963) *The Minnesota Test for the differential diagnosis of aphasia*, University of Minnesota Press, Minneapolis

Schuell, H. (1974) *Aphasia theory and therapy*, University Park Press, Baltimore

Searleman, A. (1977) A review of right hemispheric linguistic capabilities. *Psychological Bulletin, 84*, 503–28

Seelig, J. M., Becker, D. P., Miller, J. D., Greenberg, R. P., Ward, J.

D. and Choi, S. C. (1981) Traumatic acute subdural hematoma: major mortality reduction in comatose patients treated within four hours. *New England Journal of Medicine, 1*, 1245–9

Seligman, M. (1975) *Helplessness: on depression, development and death*, W. H. Freeman, San Francisco

Shapiro, I. D. C., Zernicke, R. F., Gregor, R. J. and Diestel, J. D. (1981) Evidence for generalized motor programs using gait pattern analysis. *Journal of Motor Behavior, 13*, 33–47

Shaw, L., Brodsky, L. and McMahon, B. T. (1985) Neuropsychiatric intervention in the rehabilitation of head injured patients. *Psychiatric Journal of the University of Ottawa, 10*, 237–40

Shaw, R. (1986) Persistent vegetative state; principles for the techniques of seating and positioning. *Journal of Head Trauma Rehabilitation, 1*, 31–7

Shea, J. B. (1977) Effects of labelling on motor short term memory. *Journal of Experimental Psychology: Human Learning and Memory, 3*, 92–9

Shea, J. B. and Morgan, R. L. (1979) Contextual interference effects on the acquisition, retention and transfer of a motor skill. *Journal of Experimental Psychology: Human Learning and Memory, 5*, 179–87

Sheldon, B. (1981) *Behaviour modification: theory, practice and philosophy*, Tavistock, London

Shiffrin, R. M. and Schneider, W. (1977) Controlled and automatic information processing. II: Perceptual learning, automatic attending, and a general theory. *Psychological Review, 84*, 127–90

Skinner, B. F. (1938) *The behaviour of organisms*, Appleton-Century-Crofts, New York

Smith, D. S., Goldenberg, E., Ashburn, A., Kinella, G., Sheikh, K., Brennan, P. J., Meade, T. W., Zutshi, D. W., Perry, J. D. and Reeback, J. S. (1981) Remedial therapy after stroke: a randomised controlled trial. *British Medical Journal, 282*, 517–20

Smith, R. M., Fields, F. R. J., Lennox, J. L., Morris, H. O. and Nolan, J. (1979) A functional scale of recovery from severe head trauma. *Clinical Neuropsychology, 1*, 48–50

Spiral series (Stories and plays by various authors), Hutchinson, London

Staats, A. W. (1968) *Learning, language and cognition*, Holt, Rinehart and Winston, New York

Stein, J. F. (1985) The control of movement. In Coen, C. W. (ed.), *Function of the brain*, Oxford University Press, Oxford

Stein, J. F. (1986) The role of the cerebellum in the visual guidance of movement. *Nature, 323*, 217–21

Stelmach, G. E. and Diggles, V. A. (1982) Control theories in motor behavior. *Acta Psychologica, 50*, 83–105

Stern, J. M., Melamed, S., Silberg, S., Rahmani, L. and Groswasser, L. (1985) Behavioural disturbance as an expression of severity of cerebral damage. *Scandinavian Journal of Rehabilitation Medicine Supplement, 12*, 36–41

Stern, P. H., McDowell, F., Miller, J. M. and Robinson, M. (1970) Effects of facilitation exercise techniques in stroke rehabilitation.

Archives of Physical Medicine and Rehabilitation, 51, 526–31

Storey, P. B. (1970) Brain damage and personality change after sub-arachnoid haemorrhage. *British Journal of Psychiatry, 117,* 129–42

Storey, P. (1981) *Some psychological and emotional problems after head injury,* Headway Publications, Nottingham

Tarpley, H. D. and Schroeder, S. R. (1978) Comparison of DRO and DRI on rate of suppression of self-injurious behaviour. *American Journal of Mental Deficiency, 84,* 188–94

Taub, E. and Berman, A. J. (1968) Movement and learning in the absence of sensory feedback. In Freedman, S. J. (ed.), *The neuropsychology of spatially oriented behavior,* Dorsey Press, Homewood, Illinois

Taylor-Sarno, M. L. (1965) A measurement of functional communication in aphasia. *Archives of Physical Medicine and rehabilitation, 46,* 101–7

Teasdale, G. and Jennett, B. (1974) Assessment of coma and impaired consciousness: a practical scale. *Lancet, ii,* 81–4

Terzuolo, C. A. and Viviani, P. (1979) The central representations of learned motor patterns. In Talbott, R. E. and Humphrey, D. R. (eds), *Posture and movement,* Raven Press, New York

Thomas, E. J. (1968) Selected sociobehavioural techniques and principles: an approach to interpersonal helping. *Social Work, 13,* 12

Thomsen, I. V. (1974) The patient with severe head injury and his family — a follow-up study of 50 patients. *Scandinavian Journal of Rehabilitation Medicine, 6,* 180–3

Tizard, B. (1959) Theories of brain localization from Flourens to Lashley. *Medical History, 3,* 132–45

Trower, P., Bryant, B. and Argyle, M. (1978) *Social skills and mental health,* Methuen, London

Turvey, M. T. (1977) Preliminaries to a theory of action with reference to vision. In Shaw, R. and Bransford, J. (eds), *Perceiving, acting and knowing: towards an ecological psychology,* Laurence Erlbaum, Hillsdale, New Jersey

Tyerman, A. D. and Humphrey, M. E. (1986) Self-concept change following severe head injury. Paper presented to Headway International Conference, London

Ullman, P. and Krasner, L. (1969) *A psychological approach to abnormal behaviour,* Prentice-Hall, Englewood Cliffs, New Jersey

Van Zomeren, A. H. and Deelman, B. G. (1978) Long-term recovery of visual reaction time after closed head injury. *Journal of Neurology, Neurosurgery and Psychiatry, 41,* 452–7

Van Zomeren, A. H., Brouwer, W. H. and Deelman, B. G. (1984) Attentional deficits: the riddles of selectivity speed and alertness. In Brooks, N. (ed.), *Closed head injury: psychological, social and family consequences,* Oxford University Press, Oxford

Wade, D. T., Skilbeck, C. E., Hewer, R. L. and Wood, V. A. (1984) Therapy after stroke: amounts, determinants and effects. *International Rehabilitation Medicine, 6,* 105–10

Warren, S. A. and Burns, N. R. (1970) Crib confinement as a factor in repetitive and stereotyped behaviour in retardates. *Mental Retardation, 8*, 25–8

Warrington, E. K. (1981) Neuropsychological studies of verbal semantic systems. *Philosophical Transactions of the Royal Society of London, B, 295*, 411–23

Watts, C., Cox, T. and Robinson, J. (1983) Morningness eveningness and diurnal variation in self-reported mood. *Journal of Psychology, 113*, 251–6

Webster, D. R. and Azrin, N. H. (1973) Required relaxation: a method of inhibiting agitative-disruptive behaviour of retardates. *Behaviour Research and Therapy, 11*, 67–79

Wechsler, D. (1945) A standardised memory scale for clinical use. *Journal of Psychology, 19*, 87–95

Weddell, R., Oddy, M. and Jenkins, D. (1980) Social adjustment after rehabilitation: a two-year follow-up of patients with severe head injury. *Psychological Medicine, 10*, 257–63

West, D. R., Deadwyler, S. A., Cotman, C. W. and Lynch, G. S. (1976) An experimental test of diaschisis. *Behavioural Biology, 22*, 419–25

White, G. D., Neilson, G. and Johnson, S. M. (1972) Time-out duration and the suppression of deviant behaviour in children. *Journal of Applied Behaviour Analysis, 5*, 111–20

Whiting, S., Lincoln, N. B., Bhavani, G. and Cockburn, J. (1985) *Rivermead Perceptual Assessment Battery*. NFER-Nelson, Windsor, Berks

Wilson, B. and Moffat, N. (1984) *Clinical management of memory problems*, Croom Helm, London

Wilson, B., Cockburn, C. and Baddeley, A. (1985) Rivermead Behavioural Memory Test. Thames Valley Test Co., Reading

Winstein, C. J. (1987) Motor learning considerations in the domain of stroke rehabilitation. In Duncan, P. W. and Badke, M. B. (eds), *Motor deficits following stroke*, Year Book Publishers, Chicago

Wolpe, J. (1982) *The practice of behaviour therapy*, Pergamon Press, Oxford

Wood, R. Ll. (1984) Behaviour disorders following severe brain injury: their presentation and management. In Brooks, D. N. (ed.), *Closed head injury: psychological, social and family consequences*, Oxford University Press, Oxford

Wood, R. Ll. (1986a) A neurobehavioural approach in the rehabilitation of severe brain injury. In Mazzuchi, A. (ed.), *Neuropsychological rehabilitation*, I. L. Mulino, Italy

Wood, R. Ll. (1986b) Clinical constraints affecting human conditioning. In Davey, G. (ed.), *Human conditioning*, John Wiley, Chichester

Wood, R. Ll. (1987) *Brain injury rehabilitation: a neurobehavioural approach*, Croom Helm, London

Wood, R. Ll. and Eames, P. (1981) Behaviour modification in the rehabilitation of severe brain injury. In Davey, G. (ed.), *Applications of conditioning theory*, Methuen, London

Wu, Y. and Voda, J. A. (1985) User friendly communication board for nonverbal, severely physically disabled individuals. *Archives of Physical Medicine and Rehabilitation, 66,* 287–8

Ylvisaker, M. (1985) *Head injury rehabilitation: children and adolescents,* College Hill Press, San Diego

Young, G. C., Collins, D. and Hren, A. (1983) Effect of pairing scanning training with block design training in the remediation of perceptual problems in left hemiplegia. *Journal of Clinical Neuropsychology, 5,* 201–12

Young, J. A. and Wincze, J. P. (1974) The effects of reinforcement of compatible and incompatible behaviours on self-injurious and related behaviours of a profoundly retarded female adult. *Behaviour Therapy, 6,* 614–23

Yu, J. (1976) Functional recovery with and without training following brain damage in experimental animals: a review. *Archives of Physical Rehabilitation Medicine, 57,* 38–41

Yu, J. (1983) Animal models of recovery with training after central nervous system lesions. *International Rehabilitation Medicine, 4,* 190–4

Index